An Introduction to Cluttering

T0372797

An Introduction to Cluttering explores the speech disorder of cluttering, offering concrete, evidence-based methods for its diagnosis and treatment.

Cluttering is a globally recognized communication disorder, yet it is often poorly understood. This book presents a historical overview of the efforts of pioneers in the field to demystify the cluttering disorder, before introducing the aetiology and symptoms of cluttering from several perspectives: physiological, psycho-linguistic, neurological, social, affective, and cognitive. It also provides an in-depth discussion of the identification, differential diagnosis, and assessment of cluttering, using current and advanced diagnostic procedures before explaining the rationales and unique, innovative procedures for evidence-based treatments of cluttering. Engaging practical examples and theory boxes are featured throughout the book.

Providing effective and user-friendly procedures for cluttering diagnosis and intervention, this book is an essential read for all current and future speech and language therapists.

Yvonne van Zaalen is a professor, researcher, clinician, and in-demand speaker, whose contributions to understanding cluttering, its assessment, differential diagnosis, and treatment have made her one of the world's leading experts in the field. Dr. van Zaalen is a Professor of Relational Care at the Hague University, the Netherlands, and is a recipient of the Deso Weiss Award for Excellence in the Field of Cluttering, sponsored by the Stuttering Foundation.

Isabella Reichel is a professor at Touro University, USA. She is a Board-Certified Specialist in Fluency Disorders, a Fellow of the American Speech-Language-Hearing Association, and a recipient of the Deso Weiss Award for Excellence in the Field of Cluttering, sponsored by the Stuttering Foundation.

An Introduction to Cluttering

A Practical Guide for Speech-Language Pathology Students, Clinicians, and Researchers

Yvonne van Zaalen and Isabella Reichel

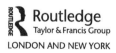
Routledge
Taylor & Francis Group

LONDON AND NEW YORK

Designed cover image: © Getty

First published in English 2024
by Routledge
4 Park Square, Milton Park, Abingdon, Oxon OX14 4RN

and by Routledge
605 Third Avenue, New York, NY 10158

Routledge is an imprint of the Taylor & Francis Group, an informa business

Published in Dutch as Praktijkboek Broddelen by Uitgeverij Coutinho 2022

British Library Cataloguing-in-Publication Data
A catalogue record for this book is available from the British Library

Library of Congress Cataloging-in-Publication Data
Names: Van Zaalen, Yvonne, author. | Reichel, Isabella, author.
Title: An introduction to cluttering : a practical guide for speech-language pathology students, clinicians, and researchers / Yvonne van Zaalen and Isabella Reichel.
Other titles: Praktijkboek broddelen. English
Description: Abingdon, Oxon ; New York, NY : Routledge, 2024. | Includes bibliographical references and index.
Identifiers: LCCN 2023050463 (print) | LCCN 2023050464 (ebook) | ISBN 9781032607887 (hardback) | ISBN 9781032607870 (paperback) | ISBN 9781003460558 (ebook)
Subjects: LCSH: Cluttering (Speech pathology) | Cluttering (Speech pathology)—Treatment.
Classification: LCC RC424.5 .V3613 2024 (print) | LCC RC424.5 (ebook) | DDC 616.85/5—dc23/eng/20240117
LC record available at https://lccn.loc.gov/2023050463
LC ebook record available at https://lccn.loc.gov/2023050464

ISBN: 978-1-032-60788-7 (hbk)
ISBN: 978-1-032-60787-0 (pbk)
ISBN: 978-1-003-46055-8 (ebk)

DOI: 10.4324/9781003460558

Typeset in Sabon
by Apex CoVantage, LLC

Contents

Editorial

It has been over ten years since *Cluttering: A (mis)understood disorder* was published (Van Zaalen & Winkelman, 2009). In the meantime, a lot has happened in the world, in healthcare, speech-language pathology, and the field of cluttering. No matter how well-known the term "cluttering" is now for speech therapists, it is often an unknown concept for ordinary people. "Hesitating" and "babbling" are often better understood on the street than the word "cluttering". Even Google automatically translates the word "cluttering" to "junk", referring to the accumulation of too much "stuff" (also called cluttering in English).

This does not make it any easier for people with cluttering. They have a speech issue, but do not know how to name it, and therefore cannot understand it. In 1717, the Swiss physician David Bazin was perhaps the first in modern times to describe cluttering, in Latin: *Dissertatio medica inauguralis de lingua et ejus vitiis morbosis* (Luchsinger, 1951, 1963). It was only through the publications of the Austrian physician Deso Weiss, two-and-a-half centuries later, that the term cluttering became more widely recognized (Weiss, 1964, 1968).

Until then, cluttering did not appear as a separate disorder and remained not generally understood until the end of the twentieth century. Myers (1996) found that between 1964 and 1996, only 36 articles on cluttering appeared in the international literature. Around the year 2000, a variety of symptoms that were difficult to categorize were increasingly attributed to cluttering, but there was still no clear, universally accepted understanding of the nature of cluttering. As more about cluttering has been published in North America and Europe over the past two decades, the condition has been more widely recognized. Given that cluttering has only recently received more recognition, compared to other communication disorders, it is not surprising that cluttering was often presented as the "orphan" of speech-language pathology.

It seems, however, that cluttering is gradually finding a niche within the family of communication disorders. This book certainly contributes to that. There are not many books on cluttering, and texts on cluttering are usually full of references to the many controversies surrounding the disorder. This can be confusing or puzzling for practicing speech therapists. In this book, Yvonne van Zaalen and Isabella Reichel provide clarity. They consider cluttering to be a rate-based communication disorder characterized by an excessive number of typical disfluencies or reduced speech intelligibility, and pauses that are too short. The authors arrive at their conclusions based on their extensive literature review, scientific research, and clinical experience. They have come up with clear suggestions, ideas, and recommendations for both assessment and treatment. This practical orientation and the extent of detail are truly unique to a disorder like cluttering. For speech therapists, this book is a rich source of inspiration that can provide guidance in their interventions for people with cluttering. Some of the suggestions and recommendations included are supported by research; others are mainly practice-oriented and are still waiting for further research to be carried out. As such, this book invites discussion on how best to move forward from this point, giving inspiration to researchers in the field. The integration of previous knowledge, the personal perspectives of the authors, and the questions raised for future research render this book a fascinating read for anyone who deals with communication disorders.

Foreword

In 2009 and 2014 the first and second editions of the book *Cluttering: A (mis)understood disorder* were published. I (Yvonne van Zaalen) wrote this book in collaboration with Coen Winkelman. Both editions were adopted in courses in the Netherlands, Europe and far beyond. I thank Coen for his friendship and cooperation in these versions.

An Introduction to Cluttering, written with Isabella Reichel, describes the latest advances in the field of cluttering, with all their positive and negative aspects. Any speech therapist can treat cluttering effectively, provided they opt for objective assessment and carefully performed differential diagnosis. The theoretical underpinnings, diagnostic tools, intervention planning, and therapeutic suggestions are based on current scientific research and on the authors' extensive clinical experience (practice-based evidence). Throughout the book, case examples have been used to clarify and enliven the message.

This book not only provides speech therapists with a theoretical framework for understanding the multifaceted phenomenon of cluttering; more importantly, it helps people with cluttering, their families, speech therapists, and other professionals by offering clinical insights into the nature, diagnosis, and successful treatment of this often overlooked, misdiagnosed but fascinating communication disorder.

Yvonne van Zaalen, PhD
Isabella Reichel, EdD

Part 1
Theoretical background

1 History, definition, and explanatory models

1.1 What is cluttering?

For centuries, physicians and speech therapists overlooked cluttering as an insignificant condition. It was only after the German Adolf Kussmaul (1877) and later the Austrian Deso Weiss (1964) drew attention to this unique phenomenon that the disorder began to receive more recognition. However, this recognition was mostly limited to Europe until the end of the 20th century. In the first two decades of the 21st century, cluttering has become widely recognized in many countries around the world. People with cluttering (PWC) are now cared for by speech therapists who specialize in the research and treatment of cluttering.

There are two subtypes of cluttering, one in which poor intelligibility is the primary issue and the other in which an excessive number of typical disfluencies interfere with the listener's comprehension. In both cases, the

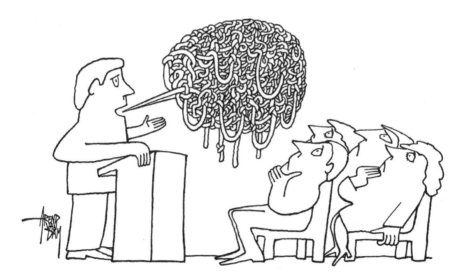

Figure 1.1 Cluttering (© Arend van Dam)

DOI: 10.4324/9781003460558-2

intended message is either not conveyed or is not understood correctly. Often, PWC are not aware of their poor intelligibility or excessive typical disfluencies during their speech, due to inadequate speech monitoring and their difficulty adjusting their articulatory rate to the linguistic demands of the moment.

There is a global consensus that PWC tend to speak at an excessively high and/or variable articulatory rate, resulting in a mismatch between the planning of speech and language and the rate of communication. The high rate of speech observed in PWC is not limited to their speaking alone but also extends to their thinking and acting due to the central organization of human behavior, particularly in the basal ganglia.

Over the past 150 years, cluttering has been defined numerous times, with many definitions simply serving as descriptions of the phenomenon. We will examine the directions in which the cluttering definition has advanced throughout recent years in Section 1.3.

1.2   International Cluttering Association

It is common to hear PWC say that they are not stuttering, but rather engaging in a form of mumbling when communicating. These individuals observe that "listeners complain that my speech is very fast and unintelligible, and I want them to stop whining about my speech." (See Figure 1.1.) Now, such people can be helped by speech therapists around the world, especially after the International Cluttering Association (ICA) was created in 2007. Among the main goals of the ICA are the creation of a platform for future research and the promotion of a consensus on the diagnosis, nature, and treatment of cluttering across continents, countries, and regions where individuals seek help for this disorder (Reichel, Scaler Scott & Van Zaalen, 2012; Reichel & Draguns, 2011; Reichel, 2010). It would be beneficial for the ICA Board to welcome more cluttering specialists to conduct more research and to provide additional innovative and successful cluttering interventions throughout the world.

1.3   Cluttering and definitions

Deso Weiss (1964, p. xi) identified cluttering as a significant disorder, not only affecting speech but also language and communication in general. Due to its heterogeneous nature, cluttering has been defined in various ways (Op 't Hof & Uys, 1974), with many definitions describing the symptoms of the condition rather than providing a clear, unified definition. This lack of consensus on the definition of cluttering has impeded research and the development of effective clinical procedures, as noted by St. Louis (1992) and Bakker (1996).

David Ward (2018) proposed the term "cluttering spectrum behavior" (CSB) to describe individuals exhibiting cluttering symptoms but not meeting the criteria for a cluttering diagnosis. Kenneth St. Louis (2007, p. 299), in collaboration with several other researchers, has dedicated years of work toward developing a descriptive definition of cluttering which is called the Lowest Common Denominator (LCD), which has been accepted by the ICA. A causal definition of cluttering was proposed by Yvonne Van Zaalen (2009), which was also approved by the ICA. This definition described cluttering as a fluency disorder characterized by an individual's inability to adjust their speech rate to the linguistic and motor demands of the moment. This causal definition was modified in 2022 by van Zaalen and Reichel. While the major principles of the 2009 definition remain unchanged, the essential update of the 2022 definition highlights the fact that cluttering is not considered a fluency disorder but rather a communication disorder, in which a person has difficulty adjusting their speech rate to the specific components of language at the moment of speech. This definition provides the opportunity to differentiate between syntactic and phonological subtypes of cluttering by ascertaining which component of language is not properly adjusted to a person's speech rate. This current working definition of cluttering reflects a new understanding of cluttering and is presented below.

> Cluttering is a communication disorder in which a speaker is not able to adjust the articulatory rate to the semantic, syntactic, morphological, pragmatic, and phonological demands of the moment. The individuals with cluttering who present with difficulties in adjusting their articulatory rate to the mainly semantic, syntactic, and/or pragmatic demands of the moment demonstrate syntactic cluttering. The most common symptom of syntactic cluttering is an excessive number of typical disfluencies. The individuals with cluttering who present with difficulties in adjusting their articulatory rate to the phonological and/or morphological demands of the moment demonstrate phonological cluttering. The most common symptoms of phonological cluttering are reduced speech intelligibility due to telescoping and coalescing and/or abnormal pause duration and/or abnormal syllable stress (Van Zaalen & Reichel, 2022).

The following empirical findings support the transition to identifying cluttering as a communication disorder as opposed to a fluency disorder.

Using functional magnetic resonance imaging (fMRI), Van Zaalen et al. (2009) identified a potential problem in the basal ganglia, which aligns with the findings of Per Alm, who suggests that rate control issues in cluttering originate from the basal ganglia system (Alm, 2011). Ward et al. (2015) supported this claim with the suggestion of a neurological link between cluttering and subcortical functioning and connectivity based on fMRI research. While Bóna & Kohári (2021) observed timing differences in the articulation rate in cluttering, no specific peculiarities in speech rhythm could be identified. These findings also prove many experts' belief that cluttering is not a fluency disorder.

1.3.1 *Cluttering in other languages*

In recent years, cluttering has been referred to in various ways in different languages. Although some of the terms for this condition have been in use for a while, new names for cluttering are still emerging in different countries as awareness of the condition continues to increase worldwide. Table 1.1 provides an overview of cluttering terminology in different languages. As the definition of cluttering has become more refined in the last three decades, more professional organizations are adopting the term "cluttering" if their previous terminology does not fully capture the essence of the disorder. For speech therapists who work with multilingual people with cluttering, knowledge of the terminology for cluttering in other languages can be helpful.

Table 1.1 Cluttering terminology in different languages

Language	Word for cluttering	Language	Word for cluttering
Arabic	إعتلاج الكلام	Indonesian	groyok
Chinese	yu shu zhang ai	Italian	tartagliare
Dutch	broddelen	Latin	tumultus sermonis, agitophasia, tachyphemia, en paraphasia praeceps
English	cluttering	Norwegian	løpsk tale
Estonian	cluttering	Polish	geitkot, mova bezladna
Finnish	sokkelus	Brazilian Portuguese	taquifemia
French	bredouillement, balbutiement, bafouillement, anonnement	Russian	Battarism, poltern, cluttering
German	Gaxen, Poltern, Bruddeln	Spanish	Tartajeo
Hebrew	דִּבּוּר חוֹטֵף	Swedish	Skenande tal
Hungarian	Hadards	Turkish	Hızlı konuşma

1.4 Main characteristics of cluttering

Op 't Hof and Uys (1974) and Langová and Morávek (1970) have acknowledged that identifying cluttering in individuals has been challenging since many people who exhibit cluttering behaviors do not consider their speech to be problematic and do not seek professional help. Additionally, Wolk (1986) has described the frequent disagreements among professionals regarding the symptoms of cluttering which further complicates its diagnosis. To accurately diagnose cluttering, St. Louis (1992) has emphasized the importance of being specific in identifying its symptoms and distinguishing it from other conditions. According to the principles of evidence-based practice and practice-based evidence, PWC typically exhibit an articulatory rate that is perceived as excessively fast and/or irregular, in combination with one or more of the three main characteristics as described by St. Louis et al. (2007).

1. Impaired speech intelligibility due to telescoping or coalescence
2. High frequency of typical disfluencies
3. Atypical pauses

These characteristics of cluttering are described by various authors, including Daly (1986), Daly & Burnett (1996), Damsté (1984), Gutzmann (1893), Mensink-Ypma (1990), Myers et al. (2018), Myers & Bradley (1992), Scaler Scott (2020), Scaler Scott et al. (2022), St. Louis (1992), St. Louis et al. (1996, 2007), Van Zaalen (2009, 2022), Van Zaalen et al. (2009, 2009b, 2011a, 2011b), and Weiss (1964). One of the notable features of cluttering is that its symptoms typically manifest when the speaker uses a fast and/or irregular articulatory rate and produces structures with high linguistic complexity, particularly when the speaker is not sufficiently focused on their speech output. However, when PWC become more conscious of their speech, their symptoms are no longer audible or visible for a period of time. Section 1.5.3 will provide an explanation for the impact of the attention of PWC on speech. After discussing the high and/or irregular articulatory rate, the following sections will provide a more detailed explanation of the three main characteristics of cluttering.

1.4.1 A fast and/or irregular articulatory rate

The primary concern regarding an articulatory rate that is excessively fast, or irregular is not the number of syllables per second but whether speakers are able to adjust their speaking rate to the time required for formulating language. Generally, fluent speakers slow down their speech rate when communicating in more complex linguistic contexts or when faced with challenging situations and speak a little faster in easier contexts or when discussing emotionally loaded topics. Despite this, the speech of PWC is often perceived as too fast and/or irregular. However, Bakker et al. (2000) have suggested that if the number of syllables produced is used to calculate speech rate, as determined through spectrograms, the rate of PWC falls within the normal range of syllables per second, although it may be perceived as very fast (St. Louis et al., 2007). It is noteworthy that Bakker et al.

examined the syllables actually produced rather than the intended sylla-bles in the message. The discrepancy between objective measurements and subjective listener judgments is primarily due to the excessive number of typical disfluencies, abnormal prosody, and errors in pausing and word structure. The speech production of PWC is so impaired that it affects the processing time of listeners, creating the perception that speech is even faster than measured.

The issues with intelligibility are caused mainly by difficulties in pho-nological planning, which involve reducing the number of syllables in multisyllabic words. This phenomenon of overcoarticulation is known as telescoping (when syllables are omitted) or coalescence (when syllables are collapsed or other errors in phonological encoding). Misunderstand-ings arise mainly due to formulation during thinking, leading to a high fre-quency of typical disfluencies and errors in pausing. PWC exhibit a higher number of disfluencies than controls, demonstrating problems in their lin-guistic formulation (Bóna, 2019).

1.4.2   *Reduced speech intelligibility due to telescoping or coalescence*

The articulatory rate is dependent on the duration of speech sounds. When producing a long sound with tension and emphasis, there must be a delay in initiating the next sound. Failure to delay adequately results in an exces-sive speech rate and abnormal prosody of speech (Alm, 2011). In the cases of telescoping and coalescence, the articulatory rate is not adjusted to the phonological demands of the moment, and there is limited time left for pho-nological encoding and motor planning.

Telescoping

Telescoping is a phenomenon in which certain syllables, usually un-stressed ones, are not articulated, as illustrated in Figure 1.2 with the pronunciation of /tescopy/ instead of "telescoping." Additional exam-ples of telescoping include /tevision/ instead of "television," and /oc-cance/ instead of "occurrence."

The word structure errors caused by telescoping (syllable omission) and coalescence, can be attributed to the speaker's limited time for pho-nological encoding of the syllables. To calculate the articulatory rate of the word "telescoping," the time needed for producing the word is divided by the number of syllables. This is because the speaker intended to generate the complete form of the word, whereas the listener hears only the version produced with telescoping.

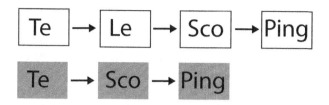

Figure 1.2 Example of telescoping (pronunciation and intended pronunciation)

Coalescence

Overcoarticulation occurs when, for example, a speaker says /amlance/ (consisting of two syllables) instead of the word "ambulance" (with three syllables), resulting in the omission of a syllable and conflation of syllabic parts, a process known as coalescence.

Within the coalescence, a distinction is made between the fusion of adjacent syllables, such as /saret/ for "cigarette" or /spot/ for "support," and the fusion of two adjacent sounds, as with /vet/ for "sweat" or /kijen/ for "kitchen." Regarding coalescence, the following errors can be differentiated: segmentation errors, sequencing errors, and phonemic errors:

- Segmentation error: one syllable is removed and parts of syllables merge to form a syllable, as in /implations/ for "implications."
- Sequencing error: syllables are put in the wrong order, e.g., /Magadaskar/ for "Madagascar."
- Phonemic error: wrong phonemes are used in syllables, e.g., /spossible/ for "possible."

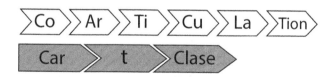

Figure 1.3 Example of coalescence (pronunciation and intended pronunciation)

1.4.3 *Excessive number of typical disfluencies*

"I want to . . . I wish . . . I had . . . but let's actually say um . . . um . . . The day of the . . . by the time I was healed, I hadn't fully recovered."

Frequent revisions, incomplete sentences, and word and sentence repetitions can present significant comprehension challenges for the listener. These disfluencies are typical and stem from the lack of adjustment of the articulatory rate to the syntactic demands of the moment, leading to insufficient time for word retrieval and planning grammatical structures. In PWC, the use of typical disfluencies during speech can provide additional time for language formulation. In fact, Bóna (2021) suggests that PWC may even interrupt their speech earlier than fluent speakers to focus on self-correction, by using typical disfluencies.

1.4.4 *Atypical pauses*

PWC tend to shorten their pauses to less than 0.5 seconds. Atypical pauses are not caused by avoidance or anticipation of stuttering (Scaler Scott et al., 2022) but by a high speech rate and a lack of inhibition, difficulties with word finding in the limited time available, hesitations, and language formulation problems. Such speech can lead to insufficient preparation for the next utterance, disturbance in breathing patterns, and difficulty in processing the message by the listener. For speakers to have enough breath to produce the next sentence, they need at least 0.5 seconds to lower the high position of the diaphragm while speaking. If the pauses are too short, speakers will have to stop again after a few words to replenish their breath supply.

The phenomenon of "being out of breath" explains why speakers take breaths in linguistically incorrect places. The lack of inhibition explains why speakers are not inclined to stop at the end of a sentence. However, providing the comment "Feel free to stop, breathing is free" can usually help clients stop this inner urge to keep going without pauses. It is necessary to provide audio-visual feedback training (see Chapter 7, Section 7.4) to develop a habit of making appropriate pauses.

1.4.5 *Prevalence and incidence of cluttering*

Understanding the prevalence of a particular disorder can aid speech therapists in identifying risk factors, planning clinical services, training professionals, and formulating educational policies (Proctor et al., 2008). However, the prevalence and incidence of cluttering are not well-documented in the literature (Van Zaalen & Reichel, 2017). Some authors have estimated prevalence rates for PWC, as shown in Table 1.2. Among children diagnosed with speech-language disorders, the prevalence of cluttering ranges from 0.4 to 11.5 percent, while combined cases of cluttering and stuttering have a prevalence of 14.8 percent. Studies that focused on differential diagnoses of fluency disorders indicate that 5 to 27 percent of PWC exhibit pure cluttering, while 13 to 43 percent of PWC in clinical settings show symptoms of cluttering and stuttering.

Table 1.2 Overview of estimates of cluttering prevalence in various populations and age groups. Some fields are blank due to an absence of data

Study	Cluttering	Cluttering-stuttering	Population Type	N
Freund in Germany (1952)	10%		Neuro-psychiatric patients with tachylalia	50
Freund in Germany (1970)		22%	Children with speech and language disorders	7227
Perello in Spain (1970)	0.4%			
Becker and Grundmann in Germany (1970 or 1971)	0.8% to 1.8%		School-aged children (7–8 years)	4984
Preus in Norway (1973)	12.7%	19.2%	Children with Down syndrome	47
Simkins in USA (1973)	11.5%		Children attending special education courses	
Preus in Norway (1981)		32%	Adolescents	256
Van Riper in USA (1982)	12%	40%	Children with fluency disorders	
Daly in USA (1993)	5%	10%	Clients with fluency disorders	
Shklovsky in Russia (1994)		33%	Clients with stuttering who entered his clinic	
Giorgieva and Miliev in Bulgaria (1996)	27%		School age and young adults with fluency disorders	15
Missulovin in Russia (2002)	1	48% (ages 12–14) 38% (ages 15–17) 31% (ages 18–53)	Patients who stutter due to organic cerebral insufficiency	
Filatova in Russia (2005)	7%	13%		
Miyamoto, Hayasaka, and Shapiro in Japan (2006)	1%	14.9 %	Special classes for children between 6–12 years of age, with speech and language disorders	208
Van Borsel and Vandermeulen in Belgium (2008)	78.9%	17.1%	Children with Down syndrome	
Van Zaalen, Wijnen, and Dejonckere in the Netherlands (2009c)	18%	43%	Adult clients with fluency disorders	54
Howell and Davis in England (2011)		17.7%	Pre-adolescents with fluency disorders at two different times	96
Van Zaalen and Reichel in the Netherlands (2014)	1.1%		Children aged 10–12	270
Van Zaalen and Reichel in Germany (2014)	1.2%		Children aged 10–12	85

According to Ward (2018), the prevalence rates of cluttering vary depending on age groups and levels of intellectual development. To analyze the distribution of the disorder, it is important to differentiate between syndromic and non-syndromic presentations of cluttering epidemiology, as suggested by Drayna (2011). In individuals with organic cerebral insufficiency, prevalence data suggest rates ranging from 38 to 48 percent, depending on age. Preus (1972) calculated a 12.7% rate of pure cluttering among individuals with Down syndrome, while Van Borsel and Vandermeulen (2008) found that 78.9 percent of this population had pure cluttering. However, caution should be taken in considering the latter figures as the diagnostic tool. The Predictive Cluttering Inventory (PCI) (Daly & Cantrell, 2006), lacks sensitivity and specificity in detecting cluttering, as pointed out by Van Zaalen et al. (2009b). Therefore, the use of the PCI in its original form is not recommended, as even its author, David Daly, acknowledges.

> The PCI-revised (Van Zaalen et al., 2009b) is recommended as a screening tool for identifying possible cluttering, consisting of ten items that differentiate cluttering from other disorders.

The lack of clarity and agreement regarding the prevalence of cluttering can be attributed to four main factors. Firstly, researchers have used different definitions to diagnose cluttering. Secondly, some studies have relied on self-reported questionnaires and subjective characteristics by simply asking people whether they thought of themselves as being PWC to diagnose cluttering without considering other factors, such as the articulatory rate and typical disfluencies, that may affect the diagnosis of stuttering or other communication disorders. This has led to the misdiagnosis of stuttering for individuals with combined cases of stuttering and cluttering. Thirdly, there was a lack of agreement as to the main characteristics and underlying mechanisms for cluttering, making a definitive diagnosis difficult. Finally, cluttering is often accompanied by other speech and language disorders and pure cluttering seems to be rare. However, a prevalence study based on clinical evaluations is now feasible given the general worldwide agreement on the main differential diagnosis and the belief that PWC have an imbalance in the basal ganglia, which prevents them from adjusting their articulatory rate to the linguistic or motor demands of the moment. Previous studies have reported rates of cluttering ranging from 1.8 percent in a German school (Becker & Grundmann, 1970) to 14.9 percent (cluttering and stuttering) in special education classes for students with speech and language disorders in Japan (Miyamoto et al., 2007).

Preus (1981) reported that 32 percent of adolescents who stutter in Norway also exhibit symptoms of cluttering. Van Borsel and Vandermeulen (2008) in Belgium found that 78.9 percent of children with Down syndrome were diagnosed with cluttering, and 17.1 percent had combined cases of cluttering and stuttering. Shklovsky (1994) in Russia reported that 10 percent of people with stuttering entering his clinic were diagnosed with cluttering. Filatova (2005) in Russia reported that 7 percent of 55 children with fluency disorders were pure cases of cluttering, and 13 percent had a mixed form of the disorder, including cluttering. Among people who stutter due to organic cerebral insufficiency, Missulovin (2002) in Russia found varying rates of cluttering depending on age: 48 percent between the ages of 12 and 14, 38 percent of adolescents between the ages of 15 and 17, and 31 percent of adults between the ages of 18 and 53. Freund (1952) in the U.S. found that 22 percent of people who stutter (PWS) also had cluttering, while Freund (1970) reported that 10 percent of neuropsychiatric patients with tachylalia were also cluttering. Daly (1993) in the U.S. found that approximately 5 percent of clients with fluency disorders had pure cluttering, and 40 percent had both cluttering and stuttering in their caseload. Despite the possibility of overlooking cluttering due to many PWC not seeking speech therapy or considering cluttering a minor condition, recent prevalence studies indicate that cluttering may be more prevalent than stuttering (Van Zaalen et al., 2011; Schnell, 2013; Van Zaalen et al., 2012). Pure cluttering may be present in 5 to 16 percent of the disfluent population, according to some experts (Bakker et al., 2005; St. Louis & McCaffrey, 2005). Prevalence rates of cluttering vary across age groups.

A prevalence study using St. Louis et al. (2007) and Van Zaalen (2009) definitions found that 2.3 percent of a group of randomly selected Dutch children aged 10 to 12 (N = 393) and 2.8 percent of a group of British students exhibited cluttering (Van Zaalen et al., 2011). These findings suggest that cluttering is more prevalent in adolescents and young adults than stuttering (Van Zaalen & Reichel, 2019). More research is needed in different languages to confirm this suggestion.

1.4.6 Etiology

Although neurological symptoms are rare in people who clutter, an organic etiology of cluttering is often hypothesized. Studies in the 1960s reported abnormal patterns in electroencephalogram (EEG) tests, which were attributed to incomplete central nervous system maturation, hemisphere dominance problems, or abnormal central auditory processing (Langová & Morávek, 1964). Researchers and therapists have concluded that cluttering is frequently observed to have a hereditary origin. Seeman (1965) reported a case of four generations in a family where 16 out of 18 members had cluttering.

When discussing the prevalence of 85 to 90 percent of family members in children with cluttering (see Section 1.2), St. Louis et al. (2007) emphasized that cluttering occurs mainly in families where many relatives have speech or language difficulties or stuttering. According to Luchsinger and Arnold (1970), cluttering is more common in men than in women by a ratio of four to one. Although this finding has not been replicated in other studies, therapists in the Netherlands and Norway who were consulted confirmed this ratio. The male-female ratio is another indication of a genetic cause of cluttering. However, it is necessary to conduct further research to determine whether this ratio is also observed in a population using the current definition of cluttering by St. Louis et al. (2007) and by the authors of this book.

Van Zaalen (2009) proposed that an inhibition problem in the basal ganglia may be the cause of the repeated production of word and non-word sequences, based on an fMRI study. The basal ganglia is a collection of nuclei located on both sides of the thalamus, with the corpus striatum being the largest group of nuclei comprising the nucleus caudate, putamen, globus pallidus, and nucleus accumbens. The substantia nigra is another core component of the basal ganglia. Earlier studies by Seeman (1970) and Lebrun (1996) investigated the role of the basal ganglia in cluttering. Seeman contrasted the symptoms of cluttering with other neurological disorders and concluded that cluttering is caused by an impairment in the basal ganglia system. At the same time, Lebrun noted that cluttering symptoms usually manifest themselves after damage to the basal ganglia system, as seen in Parkinson's disease. Alm (2011) and Ward et al. (2015) suggested that hyperactivation and dysregulation of the medial frontal cortex may also be an underlying mechanism in cluttering, with these processes being secondary to the disinhibition of the basal ganglia circuits due to a hyperactive dopamine system. The supplementary motor area (SMA) proper, together with the basal ganglia, and the cerebellum control the timing of articulatory movements and therefore the speech rate. In fluent speakers, speech production is controlled at different levels, mainly through auditory connections to the anterior cingulate cortex (ACC) and the SMA.

> Functions associated with the ACC and SMA are (1) Drive, motivation and initiation of action; (2) Inhibition of impulses; (3) Attention; monitoring and correction of behavior; (4) Planning of sequential behavior; (5) Selection of words and word-forms and (6) Execution and timing of sequential behavior (Alm, 2011, p.21).

Due to a lack of inhibition in the basal ganglia, PWC have a tendency to initiate speech prior to the completion of the language formulation phase and/or before the speech plan is adequately prepared. According to Van Zaalen (2009), the impulses for motor activity after speech production in PWC are not sufficiently inhibited or erased. As a result, syllables (and sometimes entire words) may become "stuck," leading to a negative impact on the execution of the remainder of the sentence. Examples highlighting this phenomenon are provided below.

(Retelling The Wallet Story): "It was a rainy day. A young girl called her, crying 'rainy'." Explanation: A fact from the first sentence of the story is used again – and incorrectly – here at the end of the story.

PWC, as well as their family members, often report instances of inhibited behavior in other areas. This may manifest as difficulty falling asleep, heightened levels of energy, and a tendency to react impulsively. Notably, these inhibitory deficits may also impact the individual's ability to sequence activities effectively, resulting in forgetfulness or tardiness. These behaviors are likely attributable to the abnormal functioning of the ACC and SMA.

1.4.7 Signs of possible cluttering in school-aged children

Froeschels (1946) identified a significant number of school-aged children with cluttering who were receiving treatment at public school speech clinics. Likewise, Simkins (1973) estimated that 11.5 percent of special education students exhibited symptoms of cluttering. In a sample of 4,984 school-aged children, Becker and Grundmann (1970) observed a positive correlation between age and prevalence rates of cluttering. Specifically, the prevalence of pure cluttering among children 7–8 years of age was found to be between 0.8 and 1.8 percent.

Note: It should be noted that not all studies included in this chapter are based on identical definitions or the same populations. Moreover, numerous studies have centered primarily on individuals who stutter, even though there are undoubtedly speakers with cluttering who can be found within the general population.

Speech therapists typically encounter children and adults who exhibit exclusively cluttering-like speech when they present with symptoms of cluttering. Indicators of potential cluttering during early development are recognized, and if a child demonstrates one or more of the following characteristics, it is recommended that the speech therapist conduct a differential diagnostic evaluation to consider the possibility of cluttering:

Signs of potential cluttering in young children (under ten years old):

- A fast speech or articulatory rate.
- Telescoping when using multisyllabic words.
- Omitting small words (such as articles and prepositions) when reading aloud, when writing, or during auditory memory tasks.

- Semantic or syntactic errors during fast writing or speaking, although these errors disappear during slower writing or speech.
- Stuck while reading; rely on guessing while reading.
- Many errors occur while reading at a fast rate (but not at a slow rate or when sufficiently focused on reading).
- Grapheme substitutions between /b/ and /d/.

1.4.8   *Cluttering and normal development*

To date, no longitudinal studies have investigated the developmental trajectory of speech and fluency in PWC. As previously discussed, one of the key characteristics of cluttering is the inability to adjust the articulatory rate to the linguistic demands at the moment of speaking. During the school years and particularly in adolescence, there is a notable increase in the articulatory rate observed in PWC.

The mean articulatory rate increases gradually from toddler and preschool age up to pre-adolescence, as shown in Figure 1.4 However, during adolescence, there is a significant increase, with the highest mean rate observed at approximately 17 years of age. Toward the end of adolescence, there is a considerable drop in the articulatory rate, which continues into the period of menopause (perimenopause and menopause). A possible correlation between hormone balance and the articulatory rate has been suggested, but further investigation is required to validate this notion.

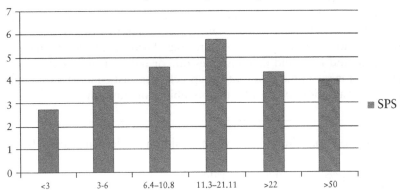

Mean articulatory rate in syllables per seconds

Age in years and months

Figure 1.4 Articulatory rate in syllables per second in children (modified figure based on unpublished data)

In adolescence and young adulthood, many individuals may first recognize that they have cluttering-like speech due to a natural increase in their speech rate. However, cluttering is typically difficult to identify in children under the age of ten since their speech rate is still too low to significantly impact fluency and intelligibility. Moreover, it can be challenging to differentiate between cluttering and language development disorders based on sentence structure errors alone. One way to differentiate between these two conditions is by comparing oral and written sentence structures since individuals with specific language disorders will make errors in both. PWC may produce errors and revisions in sentence structures only when speaking at a fast rate but not at a slower rate or when writing. Notably, the reduction in speech rate in adult-hood is a natural response to hormonal changes occurring after adolescence. If the hormonal balance is impaired in individuals predisposed to cluttering, the disorder may become chronic. Previous studies have demonstrated that cluttering manifests only when language development is at an advanced stage, and individuals have a strong urge to speak. Therefore, the late onset of cluttering is attributed to the natural increase in speech rate in adolescence and young adulthood, making it challenging to differentiate between cluttering and other childhood disorders.

The development of the speech rate in PWC is associated with an increase in self-reflection, particularly regarding their speech and appearance. During adolescence, a crucial and sensitive developmental period, individuals become more aware of speaking differently. This awareness often arises from feedback received from their social environment, such as comments like "You need to speak more clearly" or "I'm sorry, could you repeat that?"

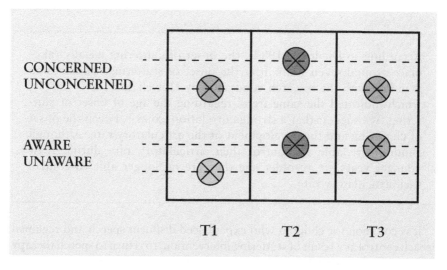

Figure 1.5 The awareness and concern of a young PWC in the transition from pre-adolescence to adolescence

However, adolescents are usually unable to identify the specific problems in their speech and subsequently struggle to adjust their speech behavior, leading to insecurity in their speech performance. This phenomenon may also contribute to the development of stuttering in PWC, as highlighted by Winkelman (1990), Ward (2018), and St. Louis et al. (2007).

A case study by Van Zaalen and Strangis (2021) provides insights into the effect of increasing the articulatory rate on speech control in adolescents who clutter. The study follows the story of Johan, a young person who was initially unaware and unconcerned about his typical disfluency at age 10.4 (T1) but became very much aware and worried about his disfluency at age 10.9 (T2) during his adolescence. See Figure 1.5. Johan was treated with audio-visual feedback training, which resulted in improved awareness of and control over his speech. A few months later, Johan was aware of his disfluencies but was no longer concerned about it.

1.4.9   *Prognosis*

Currently, there are no known longitudinal cohort studies that focus specifically on cluttering. However, based on practical experiences and anecdotal evidence, certain trends related to the age of PWC have been observed. For instance, it is often reported in the literature (St. Louis, 2011; Damsté, 1990; Mensink-Ypma (1990) that PWC may have experienced speech or language difficulties in their early years.

Nevertheless, this observation has not been systematically investigated and therefore requires further research. Longitudinal studies on children with speech and fluency problems (other than stuttering) can offer valuable insights into the development and progression of symptoms of cluttering.

> According to Diedrich (1984), the onset of cluttering usually takes place around seven years after the onset of stuttering. This finding is in line with the research conducted by Howell and Davis (2011), which indicated the same trend regarding the age of onset of cluttering. We suggest that a strong correlation exists between the onset of cluttering and the development of the articulatory rate. Although children are able to control their articulatory rate during their younger years, at an older age they are no longer able to control their articulatory rate.

It is common for children who experienced disfluent speech and regained speech control as a result of stuttering intervention, to return to speech therapy between the ages of 10 and 13. During the early years of adolescence, communication disruptions often reoccur due to natural development, with PWC exhibiting an increase in speech rate and use of more complex vocabulary and advanced syntactic constructions. As a result, their speech becomes less fluent and less intelligible. If cluttering manifests in preadolescence (10–12 years), symptoms tend to worsen during adolescence, with the increase of the articulatory rate occurring around the age of 16–17. However, the severity of cluttering may decrease after adolescence, especially if negative emotions did not develop during the period of disfluent speech or impaired intelligibility. Monitoring the articulatory rate of adolescents and teaching them to control their rate by using pauses between words and sentences is crucial. The prognosis will depend less on the increase in the articulatory rate and more on active efforts to modify speech behaviors.

Various studies have investigated non-fluent language production in older adults compared to younger adults. According to a review by Engelhardt et al. (2010), older adults produce more disfluencies across various tasks than young adults, with disfluencies mainly related to lexical retrieval problems. Disfluencies are more commonly observed within sentences rather than between them, in older adults, and no differences were observed in a sentence production task designed to assess syntactic planning. However, topic maintenance in conversation was found to be affected by age-related inhibition issues, resulting in a tendency for older adults to change the topic of conversation more frequently due to difficulty inhibiting irrelevant information. The increased number of disfluencies in older adults can be explained by slower and more laborious word finding rather than being related to inhibition problems.

It is possible that the neurolinguistic processes responsible for speech-language production gradually deteriorate with age or that the ability to adjust the speech rate to linguistic demands gradually decreases. De Andrade and De Oliveira Martins (2010) evaluated 128 individuals of both genders over the age of 60 to verify the fluency profile of older adults with respect to different fluency parameters. Speech samples were collected and analyzed based on the type of speech errors and the speech rate and frequency of speech distortions based on the analysis of 200 fluent syllables. Significant differences were observed between different age groups only in the articulatory rate, with individuals over 80 years of age exhibiting an increase in the number of speech disruptions and a decrease in speech rate. Researchers concluded that the effect of aging after the age of 80 is significant.

1.4.10 Subtyping of cluttering

Damsté (1990) suggested a classification system for cluttering based on the differences between phonological and linguistic symptoms in individuals with cluttering. This system categorizes cluttering into three types: dysarthric, dysrhythmic, and dysphasic cluttering. Ward (2018) suggested subdivisions of cluttering into motor and linguistic types. However, Van Zaalen (2009) replaced the dysarthric and motor types of cluttering with phonological cluttering, as her research revealed that individuals with cluttering have difficulties with phonological encoding rather than motor execution. The dysphasic, dysrhythmic, and linguistic forms of cluttering can be narrowed down to "syntactic cluttering" (Van Zaalen, 2009).

Syntactic cluttering

Syntactic cluttering is a type of communication disorder characterized by difficulties in grammatical encoding and word retrieval when speaking at a fast rate. This phenomenon is more likely to occur when the individual is using linguistically complex constructions, as outlined in Chapter 7, Section 7.2. The symptoms of syntactic cluttering are manifested by typical disfluencies, such as phrase and sentence repetitions, interjections, hesitations, and revisions (Van Zaalen, 2009). For instance, a person may say, "I'm very busy with my paper . . . eh thesis" instead of "I'm very busy with my thesis."

Examples of clients' experiences with syntactic cluttering

One client stated that her thought processing can be compared to a collision at a train depot, where a sudden stop causes thoughts to crash into each other. She added that overcoming the desire to remain silent after producing incoherent sentences was a challenge, as it made the speaker appear unintelligent. Another client noted that the issue became more prominent when she intended to say a particular word but ended up producing an unrelated one, which she initially considered to be normal mental dyslexia. This client wondered why she could not control her speech rate and express her thoughts coherently (Exum, Absalon, Smith, & Reichel, 2010).

Phonological cluttering

Van Zaalen (2009) classified phonological cluttering as a type of cluttering characterized by phonological encoding difficulties resulting in word structure errors, such as coalescence, telescoping, or syllable sequence errors, especially in multisyllabic words produced at a fast speech rate. This type of cluttering is more likely to occur in linguistically complex speaking situations, similar to syntactic cluttering. (See Chapter 7, Section 7.2.) An example of phonological cluttering is the production of "Probly we will teetmorrow," instead of "We'll probably meet tomorrow."

To determine whether a client's cluttering is predominantly phonological or syntactic, one of the questions on Reichel's Brief Cluttering and Stuttering Questionnaire (BCSQ) (2010) was posed as follows: "What interferes more with your communication? Planning and formulating thoughts or fast and unclear speech?" Most of the clients responded that fast and unclear speech interfered with their communication more than planning and formulating sentences, indicating that phonological cluttering interferes with clients' communication more than syntactic cluttering (Exum, et al., 2010),

Examples of clients' experiences with phonological cluttering

During episodes of cluttering, the speech of PWC is often characterized as rapid and unclear, with words flowing out in a jumbled mess without clear beginnings or endings. PWC may experience word mixing, with sentences blending together into a single verbal mass, a phenomenon that is unique to cluttering. This fast flow of speech reflects the fast rate of thoughts of PWC, which outpaces their ability to articulate them, leading to a set of associated words that may be difficult for listeners to comprehend. As a result, PWC and their listeners may be left confused by the jumbled mass of words that spills out during cluttering episodes (Exum et al., 2010).

1.5   Explanatory models of cluttering

1.5.1   *Central language imbalance*

In 1964, Deso Weiss proposed a model of cluttering as a central language imbalance (CLI), which is illustrated in Figure 1.6 and discussed in Section 1.3. Weiss's model identified a spectrum of disturbances, including delayed language development, sound errors, reading and writing disorders, disruptions in rhythm and musicality, impulsivity, and restlessness. Weiss attributed all of these problems to a central imbalance or asynchrony of language. While Weiss's model is intriguing, it fails to account for the specific problems

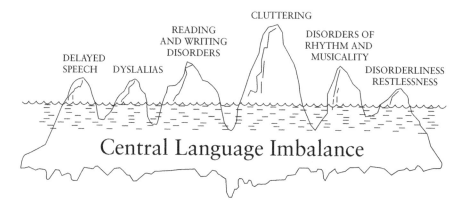

Figure 1.6 Central language imbalance

PWC have in adjusting their fast speech rate to the linguistic demands at the moment of speech. As a result, the model is no longer considered a valid explanation for cluttering.

1.5.2   Linguistic disfluency model

According to Daly and Burnett's linguistic disfluency model (1999), based on Weiss's concept, cluttering is described as a syndrome with multiple symptoms displayed simultaneously in categories such as cognition, language, pragmatics, speech, and motor skills (see Figure 1.7). Daly and Burnett believed that the diagnosis of cluttering can be made if one or more categories are affected. This model was developed to classify the different possible symptoms presented by Daly, but it is no longer used to interpret cluttering components. Daly also developed the PCI, but research has shown that it lacks specificity and sensitivity in detecting cluttering.

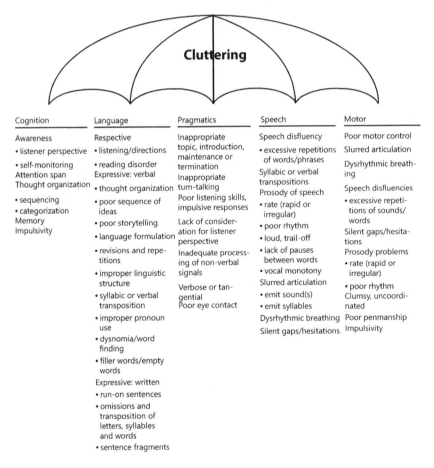

Figure 1.7 Linguistic disfluency model (Daly & Burnett, 1999)

1.5.3 Language automatization deficit model (Van Zaalen, 2009)

To understand the nature of disfluencies and speech intelligibility issues associated with cluttering, it is crucial to comprehend the language formulation processes that take place prior to language production. Van Zaalen (2009) adopted Levelt's language production model and developed her own version, which she named the language automatization deficit model. This model explains the audible symptoms observed in cluttering.

Levelt (1993) proposed a three-step process for the expression of ideas. (See Figure 1.8.) The first step involves planning the idea or message and monitoring whether it is appropriate to express it. This monitoring process is

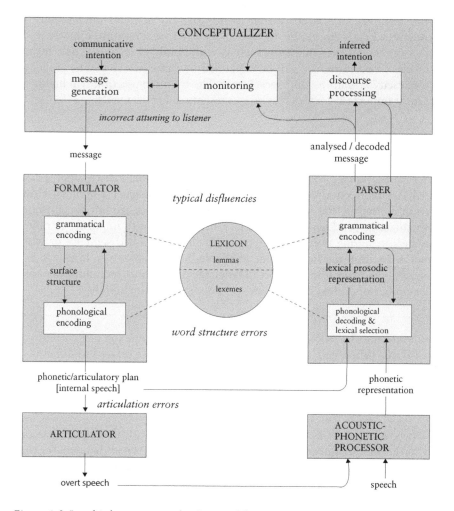

Figure 1.8 Levelt's language production model

important as it prevents people from saying things they may regret later. The second step is the formulation of the message in grammatically correct sentences. This involves constructing sentences using words from the speaker's lexicon, with each word consisting of syllables that must be produced in the correct order and manner. Once the sentences and words are planned and a motor plan is ready, the third step involves expressing the thoughts. A failure in any of these steps can result in an excessive number of typical disfluencies and speech intelligibility problems, as observed in cluttering.

Individuals with cluttering tend to speak rapidly and with an irregular speech rate, regardless of linguistic or motor demands on their linguistic system. As a result, the time allotted for completing all three stages of language production is insufficient. However, it is known that PWC can achieve fluency and intelligibility when they concentrate on controlling their speech rate. Reading aloud, especially while wearing headphones to enhance auditory feedback, has been proven to improve fluency and intelligibility in most PWC. Furthermore, the incidence of cluttering symptoms appears to be higher in relaxed environments, such as with family or friends. These inconsistencies in performance can be explained by three key elements: language automaticity, attention, and speech rate. The following section will highlight the most important factors related to these three key elements.

Language automation / dissynchronicity

A fast speech rate can lead to the production of correct sentences only if the process of language formulation is synchronous. In such cases, appropriate words are planned and produced as intended to construct sentences. However, in cluttering, the language formulation processes are not synchronous with language production due to a lack of adjustment to linguistic or motor demands, resulting in incomplete or insufficiently planned sentence or word structures within the limited time available. Such problems in language formulation processes lead to errors in language production, including an excessive number of typical disfluencies and poor speech intelligibility.

> Phonological errors and articulation errors have a lot in common. Still, the difference is clear: phonological errors are related to difficulties in planning the syllables to be produced, and articulation errors are errors in speech motor production.

There are two different types of disfluencies: typical disfluencies and stuttering-like disfluencies. Typical disfluencies are those disfluencies that most people experience when speaking, such as word repetitions (e.g., /But, but, I can do it/), interjections (e.g., /uh/, or additional pauses), phrase repetitions (e.g., /I will, I will, I will go/) and revisions (e.g., /I'm going,

I went home/). Stuttering-like disfluencies are those disfluencies character-ized by problems in motor execution, for example, sound repetitions (e.g., /b-b-butter/), prolongations (e.g., /aaaapple/) or tense pauses (e.g., /c. . .om-puter) and may be accompanied by a sense of loss of control, physical and/or emotional tension. Speech errors in cluttering are usually manifested by telescoping (e.g., /disaur/ instead of "dinosaurs") or placing the syllables in an incorrect sequence (e.g., /bli-bi-gra-fie-o/ instead of "bibliography"). Such speech errors result in problems with a speaker's intelligibility.

The occurrence of typical disfluencies can best be explained by a time-gaining effect (Howell, 2004). A person repeats that part of the message that has already been planned or adds a pause and by doing so gains time to plan the rest of the sentence. It is as if the listener can hear the speaker thinking and formulating ideas while talking. This behavior is known as maze behav-ior. (See the example below.)

> "Well, let's say I want to, um, I'm going to the, I'll drive to the zoo today."

Normally, most speakers detect and repair any speech errors they may make; however, PWC have a tendency not to identify their speech errors while they are speaking at a fast rate as they cannot direct sufficient atten-tion to this task. St. Louis et al. (2007) argue that PWC require sustained monitoring and modulation of their spontaneous speech production when discussing complex or emotionally loaded topics.

In summary, the asynchrony of language formulation and production in PWC are explained by their problems in adjusting their speech rate to the linguistic demands of their message at the moment of speech. This asyn-chrony results in an excessive number of typical disfluencies and unintelligi-ble speech.

Attention

A reliable monitoring system is essential for detecting and repairing errors in speech production. However, PWC require a significant amount of at-tention to plan sentences and words, which leaves fewer resources for other processes, such as monitoring and articulation. As a result, errors and other production problems have not been detected and remain unrepaired.

The lack of responses to speech errors or disfluencies may indicate weak monitoring skills, where control and repair processes are not initiated, due to a reduced focus.

PWC can regulate their speech production when attention is not diverted to language formulation, such as when producing nonsense syllables, retell-ing a memorized story, or describing daily activities.

PWC typically exhibit more disfluency and reduced intelligibility when speaking at home compared to a classroom setting. This phenomenon is also known as the "home disadvantage effect." It is commonly assumed that this inconsistency is due to increased stress or time pressure at school. For example, students are motivated to convey a clear message when speaking in front of a class. However, the opposite is true at home where the relaxed atmosphere reduces attention to speech and language production resulting in errors in speech and frequent disfluencies.

In cluttering, attention resources are predominantly allocated toward language formulation, leaving fewer capacities for identifying and correcting language or fluency errors, particularly during complex language formulation tasks. Therefore, cluttering is believed to be characterized by a "double deficit" involving difficulty in language formulation due to insufficient synchronicity. Subsequently, weak monitoring, as processing capacity is exhausted before the language formulation is complete. Given the inherent difficulty of formulating sentences and articulating words during the ongoing speech, monitoring speech and language production is very challenging for PWC. A dual diagnosis of cluttering with a language development disorder may be most beneficial for PWC, especially at the time of initial assessment. In Chapter 4, Section 4.7, we will describe this process for conducting a differential diagnosis.

Speech rate

According to Ward (2018), pure cluttering is uncommon, and most PWC experience rate-related problems that are caused by factors such as language automatization, language developmental issues, acquired speech and language problems, or nonspecific speech problems, like autism spectrum disorder (ASD), attention-deficit disorder (ADD) or attention-deficit/hyperactivity disorder/attention-deficit disorder (ADHD). In individuals with cluttering, language formulation difficulties are triggered by a fast speech rate. As a speech therapist, it is essential to distinguish between difficulties and disorders in PWC. Language formulation difficulties can be detected auditorily as repetitions, repairs, or mazing. These repetitions or revisions of words and phrases tend to disappear during slow speech and are noticed by PWC when they listen to their audio recordings. To eliminate the possibility of a language formulation disorder, PWC should be asked to write a story. If they can write the story without errors, a language disorder can be ruled out.

People without cluttering adjust their speech rate according to the complexity of the message. They slow down their speech when the sentence or word structure is complex and speak faster during less linguistically challenging contexts. However, PWC struggle to modify their speech rate quickly to appropriately adjust to language complexity changes.

As previously mentioned, family members of PWC often exhibit high articulatory rates and inefficient turn-taking behaviors. This can result in a fast speech rate among the family members, which can negatively impact communication for PWC. It is challenging for an individual to change speech patterns when others in the group continue to exhibit the same behavior.

PWC appear to have difficulty controlling their speech when speaking quickly. Adequate attention is required to articulate all syllables clearly. During continuous speech, PWC are unable to sustain a slower rate for an extended period (less than 40 seconds) as their attention capacity is depleted during language formulation. This phenomenon of weakening of attention is not unique to PWC, as people in general tend to lose focus after approximately 30 to 40 seconds. In PWC, the attention for speech production is typically sufficient during the initial 40 seconds and tends to decrease after about two minutes. Any change in human behavior can be maintained for a maximum of 30 to 40 seconds with sufficient focus before returning to automatic actions.

40-second rule: a person is often able to speak focused for maximum 30–40 seconds, after that automated speaking occurs and cluttering is audible. A speech therapist must assess the automated speech. For this, they need to challenge the person to speak for two minutes without interruption.

Working memory and attention capacity

Working memory is a temporary storage of information that is relevant to a task in the brain during active cognitive processes such as directing a person's current behavior, particularly in sentence formulation. Attention capacity, on the other hand, refers to the portion of working memory capacity that can be allocated to focus on additional tasks, such as the listener's response, slowing down the speech rate, or learning new behaviors. In complex language contexts, PWC utilize a significant amount of working memory for language formulation, which leads to a reduced capacity to adjust the speech rate to linguistic demands, including pragmatic aspects of language.

1.6   Monitoring in Levelt's language production model

Levelt's (1983) model of language production describes the process of monitoring and its correlation with various phases of language production (see Figure 1.8).

Conceptualizer

During the Conceptualizer phase of language production, the speaker generates a preverbal message by engaging in various processes such as formulating an intention of the message, selecting relevant information, sequencing the information, and monitoring the ongoing conversation (Olsthoorn, 2007). Internal monitoring (level 1) is the process of checking for the appropriateness and accuracy of the formulated idea. During this phase, the speaker checks whether the intended message is appropriate and useful, and whether it is worth sharing with others.

Formulator: grammatical encoding

The initial step of language production involves retrieving the appropriate words that convey the intended meaning from the mental lexicon, in the form of lemmas. These lemmas are then arranged in a syntactic framework, leading to the formation of a surface structure, which involves grammatical encoding. Selecting the precise lexical choice from a vast collection of possible alternatives is a complex process.

Formulator: phonological encoding

Phonological encoding is an essential process of speech production, involving generating a phonetic plan by selecting an abstract phonological form from lexical memory and applying it to generate articulation. During phonological encoding, segmental material is placed in a metric box that specifies the number of syllables and stress pattern to create a "phonological word with prosody." This is required to capture the prosodic framework of utterances, which can vary in different situations. Completing the syntactic surface of the utterance with the phonological word forms of the lexicon follows phonological encoding. Stress patterns and sound patterns of words are stored in the word forms section of the lexicon. The syllable structure influences phonological processing at an early stage but also remains relevant in later stages of speech production. The selected semantic representation activates the lexical-phonological representation in the phonological output, which contains the metric and segmental information of the spoken word form. This is because words can have different phonological units in different contexts.

Syllable memory

The phonetic planning process involves the retrieval of movement arrangements for commonly used syllables from the syllable memory. According to Nijland (2003), syllable memory stores and enables the reuse of commonly utilized syllables, thereby reducing the necessity for constructing motor plans repetitively. The syllable memory functions as an automatism process,

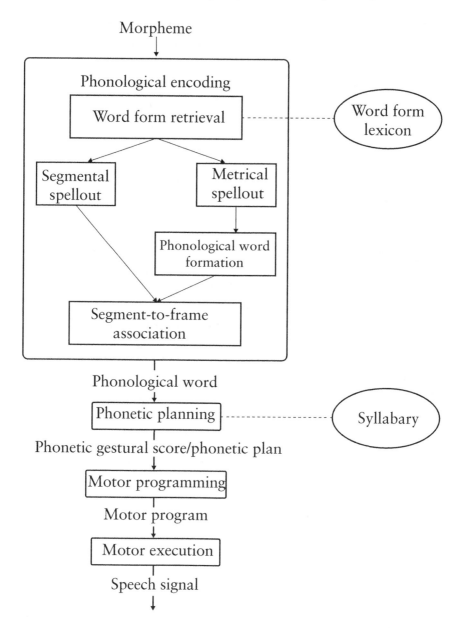

Figure 1.9 Model of speech production (Nijland, 2003)

enabling effective and effortless speech production. Nijland suggests that the consistency between the spatial and temporal characteristics of articulatory behaviors is higher within syllables than between syllables. Therefore, syllables kept in the syllable memory are likely to display more consistency.

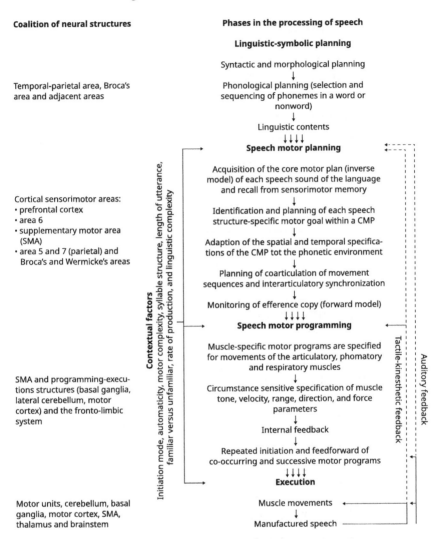

Coalition of neural structures

Phases in the processing of speech

Linguistic-symbolic planning

Syntactic and morphological planning
↓
Temporal-parietal area, Broca's Phonological planning (selection and
area and adjacent areas sequencing of phonemes in a word or
nonword)
↓
Linguistic contents
↓↓↓↓
Speech motor planning

Acquisition of the core motor plan (inverse
model) of each speech sound of the language
and recall from sensorimotor memory
↓
Cortical sensorimotor areas: Identification and planning of each speech
• prefrontal cortex structure-specific motor goal within a CMP
• area 6 ↓
• supplementary motor area Adaption of the spatial and temporal specifica-
(SMA) tions of the CMP tot the phonetic environment
• area 5 and 7 (parietal) and ↓
Broca's and Wermicke's areas Planning of coarticulation of movement
sequences and interarticulatory synchronization
↓
Monitoring of efference copy (forward model)
↓↓↓↓
Speech motor programming

Muscle-specific motor programs are specified
for movements of the articulatory, phomatory
and respiratory muscles
↓
SMA and programming-execu- Circumstance sensitive specification of muscle
tions structures (basal ganglia, tone, velocity, range, direction, and force
lateral cerebellum, motor parameters
cortex) and the fronto-limbic ↓
system Internal feedback
↓
Repeated initiation and feedforward of
co-occurring and successive motor programs
↓↓↓↓
Execution

Motor units, cerebellum, basal Muscle movements
ganglia, motor cortex, SMA, ↓
thalamus and brainstem Manufactured speech

Contextual factors
Initiation mode, automaticity, motor complexity, syllable structure, length of utterance, familiar versus unfamiliar, rate of production, and linguistic complexity

Tactile-kinesthetic feedback

Auditory feedback

Figure 1.10 The four-level framework of speech-sensomotor control (Van der Merwe & Steyn, 2018)

Weaknesses in accessing or restoring a pre-composed gestural program from the syllable memory can lead to an extension of time and less coherence of sounds in the syllable, which in turn will reduce intelligibility.

Phonological coding errors can result in telescoping, coalescence, and reduced intelligibility.

In speech production, when the words are retrieved from memory, they should be phonologically coded, during which the precise phonemes are set in the correct positions. For instance, the phoneme /d/ can be assimilated as a /t/. The phonological coding mechanism sets off the sections of the brain controlling planning articulation (Maassen & Bastiaanse, 1996), resulting in a phonetic plan. This plan ultimately is responsible for the articulator phase of language production. However, this process may be multifaceted and prone to mistakes, as illustrated in Figure 1.10 (Van der Merwe & Steyn, 2018), which outlines the several transitional stages involved in linguistic-symbolic planning, speech motor planning, speech-motor programming, and output. Despite this complexity, Levelt's model is founded on the principle of incremental sentence production (Kempen & Hoenkamp, 1987), meaning that utterances are not fully planned before articulation, but rather the speaker prepares the remaining parts of the utterance while speaking.

Phonetic plan

As previously stated, the following stage entails converting the phonological plan into a phonetic plan. This process requires identifying the spatial and temporal targets for the articulatory movements engaged in producing sounds. These targets can either be retrieved from a sensorimotor memory and adjusted to the adjacent phonemes or found from pre-existing syllable movement programs stored in the syllable memory (Nijland, 2003). Failures at this point can result in problems with accessing or restoring the correct plans for specific phonemes, leading to a groping behavior (i.e., struggling to find the correct articulation placement) during verbal tasks.

Articulator

Throughout the articulation phase, the speech plans produced in the former stages are executed as movements of the speech mechanism, leading to the production of audible speech. Problems in this phase can be presented as various speech disorders, such as stuttering, circumlocutions, or unclear speech.

Acoustic phonetic processing

Subsequently, to the execution of the intended message, the speaker becomes aware of the spoken message through auditory feedback. The accuracy of the spoken output is then examined by comparing it with the intended speech and language model. Such a monitoring process may lead to audible repairs at the syllable, word, and sentence levels, as well as repairs of the intended content of the utterance. However, PWC, due to the lack of remaining attention capacity, may experience decreased monitoring during continuing speech.

1.7 Awareness of and attitudes toward cluttering

The use of the biopsychosocial model in healthcare has been demonstrated to be highly beneficial. This model emerged during the 16th and 17th centuries with the rise of modern science, which made an apparent distinction between body and soul. The biopsychosocial model is an extension of the medical model of human functioning and reflects not only biomedical facets but also psychological and social aspects that contribute to the development of disease and influence the healing process (see Figure 1.11). In the case of cluttering, it falls under the biological factor category, along with medication and heredity. The mental health of a person with cluttering is decided by factors such as their cognitive capacity, self-confidence, and social skills. Additionally, their IQ, temperament, and past experiences within social relationships, including any traumas, influence their mental health as well.

The social component of the biopsychosocial model, as defined in the upcoming four-component model, encompasses familial, educational,

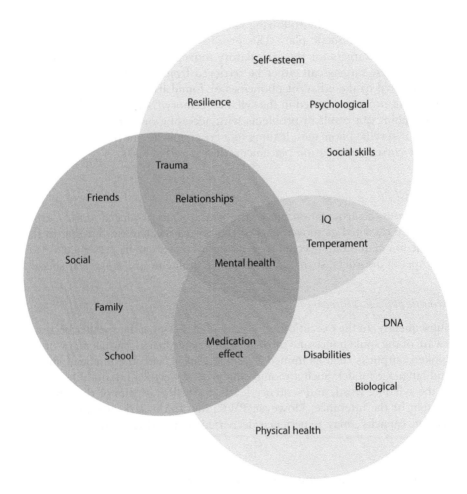

Figure 1.11 The biopsychosocial model

occupational, and social relationships and associations, and is also affected by the impact of medication. While the biopsychosocial model is useful, it requires a further explanation for the disorder of cluttering, which has been attained through the development of the four-component model.

1.7.1 Cluttering and the four-component model

The four-component model offers a description of the interaction between different communication factors in cluttering. It allows for the illustration of the various communicative characteristics of cluttering and proposes original approaches to intervention planning (see Figure 1.12). The components of cluttering have a shared influence on each other. The verbal-motor component includes a motor subcomponent and a verbal subcomponent. These subcomponents relate to all aspects of speech behavior, such as a fast and/

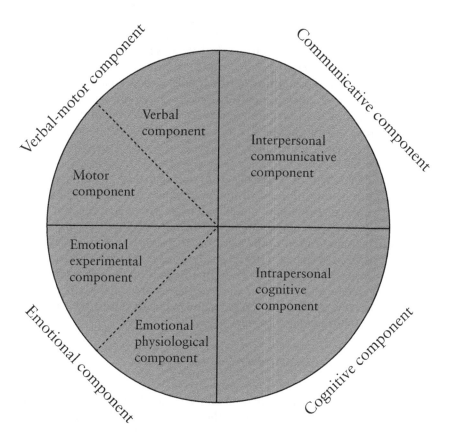

Figure 1.12 Four-component model of cluttering

or dysrhythmic speech rate, errors in word or sentence structure (e.g., telescoping, and abnormal syllable sequence), and an excessive number of typical disfluencies (e.g., word and sentence repetitions, interjections, revisions, hesitations). The motor subcomponent is related to phonological cluttering (e.g., syllable sequence and planning), whereas the verbal subcomponent is mostly related to syntactic cluttering (e.g., sentence structure, lexicon, and morphology).

The interpersonal communicative component in cluttering explains the effect of abnormal speech on the listener. Inadequate speech intelligibility and a fast exchange of communication between the speaker and listener may interfere with the listener's ability to understand the speaker. As a result, communication messages from PWC are often misinterpreted.

The emotional component of cluttering covers the impact of speech on PWC and comprises two subcomponents. The experiential subcomponent comprises the individual's past experiences with cluttering, which can result in the development of fear of communication when the person is repeatedly misunderstood. This fear is frequently disguised since the person may be unaware of its presence. Fear of communication becomes apparent when the speaker's message is not understood, and no connection can be recognized between the speaker's speech and the listener's reaction. Fear of sounds, words, or speech, however, is unlikely to arise in pure cases of cluttering. The physiological subcomponent of cluttering is displayed as a lack of inhibitory control. This makes it difficult for PWC to stop speech initiation, leading to negative effects on subsequent communication. The lack of inhibitory control does not stop or disrupt the speaker, but it is presented as physical restlessness during the speech, which may distract the listener's attention from the speaker's message.

The final component of cluttering is the intrapersonal cognitive component, which can be difficult to identify due to its discrete nature. Most individuals with normal speech have a moderately positive self-image, but PWC, due to low symptom awareness, often rate their speech positively and assign problems in communication to the listener's absence of attention. Nevertheless, their positive self-image shifts when they are faced with negative feedback from listeners. Treatment for cluttering focuses on the improvement of symptom awareness and resistance to changing speaking habits. The cognitive component is targeted both implicitly and explicitly during the cluttering intervention, as discussed in Chapters 6 and 7.

1.7.2   *Negative stigma towards cluttering in early literature*

Dalton and Hardcastle (1993) recognized that some early scientists in the field ascribed negative personality traits to PWC based on their subjective impressions. Froeschels (1946) portrayed the personality of PWC as impulsive, forgetful, careless, and chaotic at the intersection of speech and personality.

Freund (1966) described PWC as aggressive, outgoing, impulsive, uncontrolled, and hasty, with a speaking style that negatively influenced listeners, causing tension, frustration, and confusion, and requiring strong concentration to follow what the person was saying. Weiss (1964) depicted PWC as poor listeners, impatient to express their thoughts, superficial, and careless of the interests of others, and the consequences of their behavior. Weiss emphasized that PWC took the initiative in conversations and ignored the beliefs and feelings of listeners, causing annoyance due to their deficits of sensitivity and egocentricity. Weiss also stated that many adolescents who clutter communicate their anger, probably due to their generally poor school performance. PWC were presented by Weiss as worried, frustrated, short-tempered, explosive, and difficult to manage at home.

Several authors (Reichel & Draguns, 2011; Van Zaalen & Reichel, 2015; Ward, 2018) have called attention to the fact that negative personality traits have been ascribed to PWC without systematic empirical evidence. Dalton and Hardcastle (1993) argued that these negative stereotypes have not been realistically justified. Ward claims that deficient attention and self-control skills may cause inadequate listening, leading to misunderstandings and inadequate responses. Van Zaalen (2009) explains that during the moment of formulating language, PWC have reduced attention capacity to monitor their speech and respond to listener reactions. Reichel (2010) points out that the negative stigma related to cluttering may cause significant social and psychological problems. Wilhelm (2020) published a book entitled *Too Fast for Words*, in which he relates his experiences with differential diagnosis using the Cluttering Assessment Battery (Van Zaalen & Reichel, 2015), as described in Chapter 4.

Early pioneers in cluttering constructed their ideas about the personalities of PWC solely based on clinical observations, prompted by their reactions to communication difficulties. Mullet (1971) believed that pioneers in speech pathology "tried to loosen the tongue" and consequently "tried to loosen the mind" (p. 140), echoing the coercive and regular urges of their time. Nevertheless, negative stereotypes, prejudices, and stigmas towards PWC are now widely admitted as causing pain, hurt, and hatred. Such destructive attitudes persist, despite significant differences across historical periods, countries, and cultures (Reichel & Draguns, 2011).

1.7.3 Public awareness of cluttering

De Britto Pereira et al. (2008) indicate that the awareness of a communication disorder can substantially influence attitudes toward individuals with such disorders. To assess the awareness of cluttering and stuttering, an experimental version of the Public Opinion Survey of Human Attributes-Experimental (POSHA-E) was presented to a sample of the general public in four countries, namely the United States, Russia, Bulgaria, and Turkey

(St. Louis et al., 2010). The questionnaire contained layperson-oriented definitions of cluttering and stuttering.

The respondents estimated that 40 percent of individuals with fluency disorders presented with a combination of cluttering and stuttering, while 60 percent were believed to have stuttering only. Respondents from all four countries viewed cluttering and stuttering as different fluency disorders that can coincide. The most reported co-occurring syndrome in individuals with cluttering and stuttering, irrespective of age, was believed to be ADHD. Other reported co-occurring communication disorders included language disorders, articulation disorders, and unspecified conditions.

Two substantial interpretations can be ascertained regarding studies that estimate the prevalence of cluttering among disfluent speakers. Firstly, respondents are asked about the occurrence of cluttering, which is not a well-defined concept in every country. Secondly, by only examining the disfluent speaker group, a considerable number of proficient speakers, who do not exhibit disfluent speech, are excluded. This serious bias has caused lower published prevalence rates in the literature. Presently, due to increased attention to cluttering on social media, it is apparent that the number of cluttering speakers who experience problems with speech intelligibility is significantly higher than previously estimated. (See also Section 1.4.5 on prevalence.) With more people becoming aware of cluttering as a communication disorder and identifying its symptoms, public opinion is likely to change faster than in previous centuries.

To this day, a negative representation of individuals with cluttering persists among many people. When communicating with PWC, listeners may become annoyed and lose focus due to symptoms such as compulsive speaking, unclear articulation, monotonous tone, and a seemingly endless stream of speech, known as "verbal drive" (Simkins, 1973). Negative stereotypes and opinions associated with cluttering are prevalent in most cultures, but some non-Western cultures have explicit cultural beliefs that certain diseases and conditions are caused by "acts of God" or "demons or spirits," leading to further stigma (Al-Khaledi et al., 2009; Reichel & Draguns, 2011; St. Louis et al., 2007).

The POSHA-E was presented in the four countries to examine attitudes towards cluttering and stuttering, in comparison to eight other human conditions with positive, neutral, or negative associations (St. Louis et al., 2011). Participants rated cluttering and stuttering as negatively as being overweight, using a wheelchair, or having a mental illness, and more negatively than being old or left-handed. Participants linked the causes of cluttering to psychological and other factors, such as emotional trauma and tension at home. Nevertheless, these causes were believed to be less significant than they are for people who stutter.

In addition, the research performed in the four countries referred to above revealed that the respondents did not essentially reject the idea that cluttering might be caused by a virus, disease, or other supernatural factors such as "an act of God," demons, or spirits. Every country investigated demonstrated a negative stigma towards cluttering and stuttering.

Participants identified PWC as being nervous, irritable, anxious, or shy and alleged that they were not fit for jobs that require significant speaking and/or responsibility. These reactions support the negative stereotype commonly associated with people who stutter and corroborate earlier findings (Reichel & Draguns, 2011; St. Louis, 2013; St. Louis et al., 2011).

1.7.4 Awareness of cluttering in speech therapists

The awareness of cluttering and its treatment approaches have been limited to speech therapists, but currently, there has been mounting interest among educators and linguists in this disorder of speech rate. Surveys on speech therapists' awareness reveal that cluttering expertise, in general, is limited in the United States, Great Britain, Bulgaria, Australia, Belgium, Canada, Denmark, England, the Faroe Islands, Israel, Sweden, and the USA (Reichel & Bakker, 2009; Reichel, Myers, & Bakker, 2010). The responses to these surveys suggest that speech therapists lack confidence in their ability to plan, assess, and provide therapy for PWC due to inadequate academic preparation and limited access to relevant literature. This situation is changing now. There are three active Facebook pages that exist where significant questions are regularly asked and answered.

Cluttering can be treated effectively by speech therapists—generalists. Consequently, PWC can increasingly go to a speech therapist who is located geographically closer, with shorter waiting lists than the fluency therapists. In conclusion, more speech therapists now indicate that they can recognize and diagnose cluttering, and experts in the field of cluttering can be found both among stuttering specialists and among speech therapists—generalists.

1.8 Summary

This section provides a thorough overview of the various definitions and models used to explain cluttering, a disorder that was previously overlooked and misunderstood. Van Zaalen (2009) proposed a four-component model of cluttering which integrates Levelt's (1989) and Stourneras' (in Bezemer et al., 2010) models to describe the key characteristics of cluttering and its differential diagnosis with other co-existent disorders. With the advancement in the understanding of cluttering based on its theoretical frameworks, more speech therapists feel comfortable accurately diagnosing and treating this communication disorder.

Cluttering is a multifaceted disorder that may affect all aspects of communication, especially fluency and/or intelligibility of speech. When language production is simple for speakers with cluttering, their speech is fluent and clear. However, when the grammatical, morphological or phonological encoding is challenging, and the understanding of the listener may be compromised, the speech rate must be adjusted to the linguistic complexity of the utterance. Since PWC should focus their attention on formulating sentences and words, they have limited remaining attention capacity to control their speech rate. Therefore, inadequate language automatic productions result in either an excessive number of typical disfluencies or unintelligible speech.

2 Cluttering symptoms

2.1 Key characteristics

This chapter places the variety of symptoms discussed in Chapter 1 in a theoretical framework. This framework will help speech therapists to assess, diagnose, and treat cluttering.

> Diagnostic markers are measurable characteristics used to classify individuals as affected by the disorder. (Shriberg, 2003, p. 501)

Based on Shriberg's definition, measurable and strong characteristics are required to differentiate cluttering from other disorders. The phenomenon of "cluttering" involves a combination of symptoms and characteristics that manifest themselves to varying degrees in different individuals. Therefore, a diagnosis of cluttering cannot be made based on a single symptom or characteristic (Alm, 2011). People diagnosed with cluttering will have at least the following key characteristics: a perceived fast and/or irregular speech rate combined with at least one of the following symptoms:

- High-frequency of typical disfluencies.
- Excessively frequent pauses and deviations in prosodic patterns (syllable stress or speech rhythm) that are inconsistent with syntactic and semantic rules.
- Coalescence or syllable telescoping (see also Chapter 1, Section 1.4).

St. Louis and Schulte (2011) added the concept of native to the definition of cluttering when they described cluttering as "a fluency disorder wherein segments of conversation in the speaker's native language typically are perceived as too fast overall, too irregular, or both" (St. Louis & Schulte, 2011, p. 241). Assuming that cluttering is a problem in the adjustment of the speech rate where a person is not sufficiently able to adjust the speech rate to the linguistic demands of the moment, the concept of the native language is not significant for a diagnosis of cluttering. Of course, speaking in a second or

DOI: 10.4324/9781003460558-3

even a third language will slow down the speaker's rate as long as the speaker is not fluent in the new language. In such a situation, cluttering will not be evident. However, cluttering will emerge in non-native speakers, as soon as they acquire adequate proficiency in another language (van Zaalen & Reichel, 2014).

In addition to the symptoms mentioned earlier, other characteristics are often observed in PWC that are not necessarily unique to this group. These symptoms include overuse of interjections, monotonous speech, verbosity, mumbling, change in vowel clarity, and unclear pronunciation. Cluttering is only diagnosed in cases where the presence of the three above-mentioned key characteristics disrupts verbal communication, and the speech rate is too fast and/or too variable.

Not every speaker with impaired speech intelligibility or a fast speech rate should be diagnosed with cluttering. Impaired speech intelligibility, especially in young adults, as in tachylalia, can in most cases be attributed to only one of the characteristics of cluttering and not to difficulty in rate adjustment. It is common for impaired speech intelligibility and an excessive number of typical disfluencies to occur in stressful conditions. Just think back to how you spoke during your oral exams. At times like this, you do not speak of a disorder but of a reaction to a stressful situation.

This was also noted by Myers and St. Louis (1992) when they wrote that some parameters of cluttering, such as an abnormal speech rate, disfluencies, language disorders, and coarticulation, may be present independently of each other. Therefore, to diagnose cluttering, speech therapists need to know whether PWC can adjust their speech rate to the linguistic and motor demands of the moment. Part 2 of this book, "Diagnostics," provides a comprehensive description of how to diagnose cluttering.

2.2 Characteristics and symptoms

The following sections elaborate on various characteristics of cluttering and the symptoms of coexisting disorders based on the general international consensus.

2.2.1 *Too fast and/or irregular rate*

An inappropriate speech rate interferes with a person's ability to communicate effectively (Sturm & Seery, 2007). When speaking too fast, the listener is overloaded with information (Sturm & Seery, 2007) and cannot understand the message upon the first hearing, particularly because a fast speech rate affects the speaker's diction (Rodero, 2012). When assessing a speaker's rate, it is important to know the difference between the speech rate and the articulatory rate. Speech rate corresponds to the overall time used for spoken delivery of a message (Sturm & Seery, 2007). When determining the speech rate in words per minute, time spent on pauses and disfluencies is considered in calculations (van Zaalen et al., 2009). For years, scientists have considered the articulatory rate to be a good indicator of speech-motor behavior (Hall et al., 1999; Kent, 1984; Van Riper, 1982). Articulation rate is defined as the rate at which the articulators move for speech production (Chon et al., 2012). It reflects the temporal aspects of motor speech as well as motor transition ability for speech production (Chon et al., 2012) but does not take into account speaker-specific ways of conveying information, such as hesitations, pausing, emotional expressions, and so forth (Cosyns et al., 2013). The articulatory rate measured in syllables per second is a better measure of speech execution time than the speech rate measured in words per minute. The articulatory rate is the number of syllables or phonemes per second in a speech sample after removing pauses and disfluent episodes. The diadochokinetic rate (in syllables per second) investigates the (maximum) motor skills of the articulators. To avoid fatigue as a contributing factor, it is recommended to use sequences of up to 20 syllables for the analysis (Rusz et al., 2021).

> **Example of pauses that are different from sociolinguistic norms**
>
> "What I'm going with . . . my friends for dinner because . . . When I . . . do . . . don't do that, I'll be sure . . . hungry."

The speech of PWC is characterized by a high frequency of irregular and short pauses in linguistically inappropriate places. Many additional pauses significantly affect the mean speech rate in cluttering. On the other hand, cluttering is also characterized by an irregular rate. The articulatory rate is considered a starting point for comparing the speech-language productions and the critical symptom in the diagnosis of cluttering. All confounding factors should be excluded, if possible. Cluttering is about whether people can adjust their rate to the linguistic demands of the moment. Notably, all confounding factors are observed and documented during the assessment.

In the working definition of cluttering, as formulated by St. Louis et al. (2007), the observed fast and/or irregular articulatory rate is considered a mandatory feature of cluttering. St. Louis et al. note that the articulatory rate can be perceived as too fast, but when measured, the articulatory rate may be within normal limits. It is not so much about how fast a person speaks; rather, the question is whether the articulatory rate is appropriate to the demands of the person's language formulation (formulator/formulation; see Figure 1.8).

Lucio, 10 years old, has an articulatory rate of 6.3 syllables per second for storytelling, 6.7 for retelling a story, and 5.4 for quickly repeating complex words. No speech errors are evidenced. Lucio is not diagnosed with cluttering. There may be tachylalia. Lise, ten years old, has an articulatory rate of 4.8 for retelling a story and producing complex words. Lise speaks with 17 percent typical disfluencies. There may be cluttering because Lise is unable to adjust her speech rate to linguistic demands. To make an accurate diagnosis, a comprehensive assessment is needed.

While one person may communicate fluently and with good intelligibility, at an articulatory rate of more than six syllables per second, another person may manifest disfluencies or poor intelligibility. Therefore, comparing people based only on articulatory rate without considering levels of language complexity of the task presented is not recommended. More about this can be found in Part 2, "Diagnostics."

2.2.2   *Word structure*

Words are composed of syllables. The order in which syllables are sequenced can determine the word's meaning. To compose words by combining syllables, a certain amount of planning time is needed. Due to the fast rate of PWC, they often do not have enough time left for phonological planning, before the completion of phonetic planning and motor execution (Articulator; see Figure 1.8). When speakers have insufficient time to plan, they tend to make errors, including in the sequencing or structure of syllables. For example, PWC can say /magfinic/ instead of "magnificent." Also, errors in a syllable structure may occur. PWC can say, for example, /plIs/ if they mean "police." Errors in the word structure can occur due to insufficient planning time or because previously produced syllables are still present in the speaker's mind, just like a song that you keep in your head and cannot let go.

When Bertram speaks slowly, he hardly encounters syllable sequence errors. When he excitedly tells a story about his vacation in Bellport, he says, "I saw a nairbow" when he planned to say "rainbow." In telling the rest of the story, these kinds of errors increase. In other words, Bertram produces similar sequencing errors as he makes on the Screening Phonological Accuracy (SPA) test. He has a high syllable error score on the SPA test (Van Zaalen, 2011).

PWC generally manifest faster reaction times than in controls (Garnett et al., 2012). Moreover, PWC often make more mistakes than typical speakers when performing a phoneme monitoring task. These findings indicate that PWC have a self-awareness deficit that contributes to errors in speech production. For an accurate diagnosis of cluttering, it is necessary to ensure that phonetic errors that are produced by the client are related to planning errors and should be included in the assessment. Phonetic deficits should therefore be disregarded. Phonological errors are similar to those usually made by people with verbal apraxia and are found in the speech of PWC with phonological cluttering. Some experts consider these errors to be the primary symptom of cluttering (Ward, 2018). Typical for PWC are the so-called coarticulation errors. Phonetic substitutions such as /teatring/ ("treating") or /freel fee/ ("feel free"), may also be common in cluttering. PWC with phonological cluttering can have significant problems with tongue twisters, even if the speech rate is slowed down; after all, the time for planning speech is limited in PWC.

> **Tongue twister**
>
> How much wood would a woodchuck chuck if a woodchuck could chuck wood? He would chuck, he would, as much as he could, and chuck as much wood as a woodchuck would if a woodchuck could chuck wood.

During the production of such classic tongue twisters, errors like those in clients with phonological cluttering or dyspraxia of speech can be present. Therefore, the following errors may occur during the production of tongue twisters:

- Excessive coarticulation is audible, for example: /politician/ ("politician"), /plees/ ("police"), /Many think so/ ("Many people think so").
- Syllables or sounds are replaced, for example: /Magadaskar/ ("Madagascar"), /presisent/ ("president"), /tevevision/ ("television"), /tecspatle/ ("spectacle").
- Syllables are added, such as: /communicationon/ ("communication").

2.2.3 *Speech pauses*

Pauses between sentences in Anglo-Saxon languages usually range from 0.5 to 1.0 seconds (van Zaalen & Winkelman, 2014). However, pauses that are shorter than 0.2 seconds can frequently be observed in PWC. That is significantly shorter than the pauses of typical speakers. Below, we explain why pauses are so important for both the listener and the speaker.

Pauses are phonetic markers of prosodic boundaries, but the processing of previous and subsequent sentences takes place during pauses (Krivokapić et al., 2020). Pauses are essential for listeners to process and understand spoken language. During the pause between sentences, listeners can consider whether they will respond to the speaker's utterance. If the speaker makes very short pauses, the speaker will talk through the other person (inadequate turn-taking behavior) or talk when the other person wants to respond. Listeners find such behavior to be unpleasant. Communication partners of PWC regularly indicate that the person with cluttering seems uninterested in them.

The pauses are of equal importance to the speaker. Pauses provide the speaker with time to formulate and plan the sentence that follows, lower the diaphragm, and thus release the breathing tension created during the previous sentence. Pauses ensure enough oxygen to produce the subsequent sentence. The speaker who skips a pause has limited time to prepare and plan the sentence that follows. As a result of this reduced time, speakers must adjust their speech rate while speaking. Such an adjustment can manifest itself by typical disfluencies, such as revisions, interjections, or word and sentence repetitions. The following example illustrates this:

> Desirée, a 30-year-old comedienne, appears at a clinic with significant concerns about her speech performance. She is a very fast speaker and a language juggler. She spends many hours writing her skits. After the show, she talks to her fans. She finds that her fans love her but do not seem to understand much of what she is saying in her act. People who are not among her fans hate her style. They say, "This girl is so full of her own talk, but that is what it is – just talking." Desirée feels misunderstood. She often loses much of her audience due to her lack of pauses. People who try to understand her often give up because she does not give them time to understand what she is saying. The high frequency of disfluencies is interpreted by her fans as being funny. As a result, a language juggler is judged to be a clown.

Another feature of cluttering is abnormal pause placement within sentences. Because PWC speak at a fast speech rate, their pauses are usually very short, leaving them breathless in many cases. During normal language development, most people do not need to be taught where to pause in their sentences. However, the fast rate of PWC prevents them from developing this inner concept of phrasing and pauses. Identifying appropriate pause placements and sentence boundaries in a text without punctuation marks also proves difficult for many PWC. If a speaker pauses at unnatural places in the sentence, it negatively affects the comprehensibility of the message. To understand the message, the listener must process the sentence twice. That is not a problem if the speaker is silent, but PWC are inclined to continue talking.

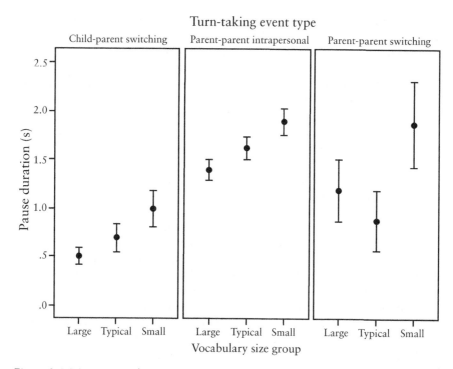

Figure 2.1 Mean pause duration (CI = 95%) in different types of turn-taking behavior, presented by lexicon group (large-normal-small)

Marklund et al. (2015) establish an average pause duration of 0.70 (SD = 1.57) during turn taking between children with normal vocabulary and their parents. During the turn-taking behavior between the two parents of these children, the pause duration was 0.88 (SD = 1.57). Figure 2.1 shows that parents of children with a limited vocabulary tend to shorten this pause duration. Family members of cluttering speakers often speak quickly, and their interaction is fast. New research can tell us whether increasing pause time during communication with family members will positively affect the comprehensibility and intelligibility of speech for PWC.

2.2.4 *Disfluencies*

The frequent occurrence of interjections and revisions has implications for the nature of fluency failures in cluttering. Although the previously prevailing view that speech disfluencies are caused by a disruption in time-dependent phonological or phonetic encoding cannot be determined in a population of fluent speakers (Eldridge, 2007), we posit that linguistic rather than articulatory problems cause an excessive number of disfluencies in PWC. This view is supported by other experts as well, including Bóna (2019), who argues that

PWC produce more frequent and longer disfluencies than controls, suggesting linguistic formulation problems in PWC. These disturbances are often referred to as "maze behavior" (Howell & Au-Yeung, 2002) or "prepares", "audible as typical disfluencies" (van Zaalen et al., 2008). As proposed by Howell and Au-Yeung (2002) in their EXPLAN model, typical disfluencies are produced to gain time to plan the next structure. The speaker repeats what was already planned and produced. The typical disfluency lasts until the planning of the next segment of the sentence is complete, and the intended structure is carried out. Therefore, the repetitions that are considered typical disfluencies are rarely tense and are produced in normal rhythmic patterns. Unlike stuttering-like disfluencies, typical disfluencies do not break up the syllable structure.

Bóna (2021) observed that thirteen-year-old and gender-matched individuals with cluttering may interrupt the speaker, contrary to what happens with fluent speakers who would try to self-repair their productions. This idea of Bóna is interesting, but it needs further research due to several considerations. Extending the formulation time, audible as typical disfluencies, often assists in arriving at grammatically correct productions.

Repetitions that are considered typical disfluencies are syllable, word, and sentence repetitions produced without tension, at a regular rate, and without additional stress (Myers & Bradley, 1992; St. Louis, 1996; van Zaalen et al., 2009, 2009b). Due to the word retrieval and a high speech rate, a high frequency of word and sentence repetitions is observed. Part-word repetitions (for example, "pa pattern") where the number of repetitions is less than two are also common in PWC. These unstressed part-word repetitions are interpreted as overt repair and are therefore counted as typical disfluencies. Stuttering-like disfluencies, such as tense word repetitions, prolongations, and tense pauses, are rare in cluttering (< 3 percent stuttered syllables) (Sasisekaran et al., 2006).

The studies of Myers and St. Louis (2007) and van Zaalen et al. (2009c) show that PWC as a group produce typical disfluencies similar to those of typical speakers. Yet sometimes the frequency of typical disfluencies is much higher in PWC. Moreover, there seems to be a difference in the frequency of disfluencies between the two subtypes of cluttering. In people with phonological cluttering, the frequency of typical disfluencies is comparable to that of fluent speakers. However, in people with syntactic cluttering, the frequency of typical disfluencies is significantly higher than in other groups. However, the question remains as to what percentage of typical disfluencies is considered to be within the normal range and is not disruptive to communication.

The frequency of typical disfluencies among fluent speakers reportedly ranges between 3.1 percent in a group of young children (De Nil et al., 2005) and approximately 9.7 percent in adolescents (Eggers, 2010; Blokker et al., 2010). In some PWC, typical disfluencies can be as frequent as 35 percent (van Zaalen et al., 2009b). PWS, on the other hand, produce, on average, less than 5 percent of typical disfluencies (van Zaalen et al., 2009b). Damsté

(1990) explains this phenomenon by suggesting that PWS even repair their speech that normally does not need to be repaired.

Note: The combination of fast speech rate, short pauses, disfluencies, and excessive coarticulation makes the perception of disfluencies even higher than the actual percentage of disfluencies as measured (Van Heeswijk, 2011). There is a great need for in-depth research into the occurrence of typical disfluencies at different levels of language complexity, in situations with and without a focus on speaking and during single or multiple attempts. By comparing people with syntactic cluttering with the entire population, we may be able to arrive at better criteria for differential diagnosis in the future.

2.2.5 Communication disorders

Communication rules are essential for a typical conversation between two or more people. For PWC, normal communication rules (pragmatics) are not always followed. Taking or giving turns can be a considerable challenge. PWC may start to talk impulsively or may keep talking without noticing listeners' reactions, partly because of their extreme focus on language formulation.

Due to insufficient speech intelligibility and/or the high frequency of typical disfluencies, stories told by PWC can be misunderstood or even completely incomprehensible. PWC are often not fully aware of why they are not understood. When asked for clarification, PWC will often repeat exactly what they just said. This can frustrate the listener and the PWC, who realize they are not understood once again. PWC who are aware of their symptoms will pronounce the words more clearly the second time. This can happen, for example, when the listener's reaction is a befuddled expression.

Introducing and maintaining a topic of conversation is often problematic for PWC. While telling a story, there is an insufficient inhibition of associations in the story, sometimes leading to the being described as "subject hoppers" or people who "jump off the hook." For the listener, this can be disruptive over time. To adequately introduce and discuss a topic, a speaker must consider the listener's knowledge. If a topic is not introduced properly, this can lead to much ambiguity, as in the example below.

Confusion due to a missing introduction

Rafael is busy talking to Giorgio to brainstorm ideas when designing a new game. While details are being discussed, Giorgio suddenly says: "That boy has been arrested and has to sit for two months." Rafael answers first, thinking about the game they are developing: "But then we also have to design a prison, and I don't know if that will still work." It takes a while for both of them to realize that Giorgo, inspired by the game's story, remembered reading in the newspaper that one of the rioters in their town had been jailed.

Weiss (1964) interprets such a lack of an adequate response to the listener as an indication of disinterest in the present conversation. Additionally, a fast communication rate of PWC makes their assessment of the listener's knowledge or information needs almost impossible. When the listener's perspective is not adequately considered by PWC, the communication turns into a monologue instead of a dialogue. However, there is no empirical evidence in the literature indicating that during communication, PWC are less able to evaluate the listener's knowledge or information needs compared to typical speakers.

2.2.6   Melodic patterns

Natural speech consists of the following aspects:

- Speech intelligibility
- Adequate vocabulary
- Use of sufficiently long pauses between language units
- Use of melodic patterns and stress (see Figure 2.2)

Impaired communication typical for cluttering can also result from abnormal melodic and prosodic patterns. These are paralinguistic parameters related to the communication described above. Several examples are given for clarification. Abnormal phrasing, fast and varying speech rate, and atypical sentence formulation can lead to rapid changes in pitch and stress patterns, monotony, and melodic monotony. The monotony makes the message difficult to understand, and the listener's concentration decreases as a result.

A frequent variation of monotony in cluttering is called melodic monotony. In monotony (see Figure 2.3), the differences in pitch are minimal (i.e., below 100 Hz within a 2–3 second sentence). In melodic monotony (see Figure 2.4), the speaker uses the same intonation pattern in each sentence,

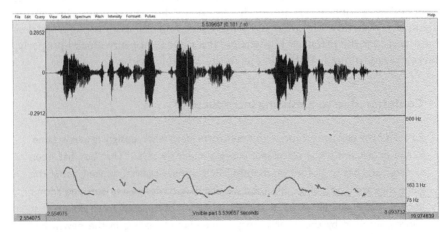

Figure 2.2 Natural melody, produced with the PRAAT software (see Chapter 4, Section 4.6.8)

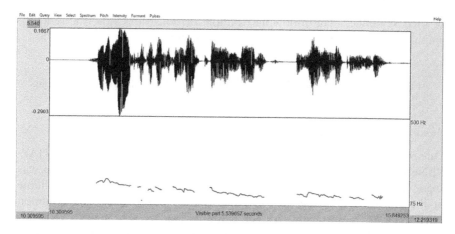

Figure 2.3 Monotony, produced with the PRAAT software

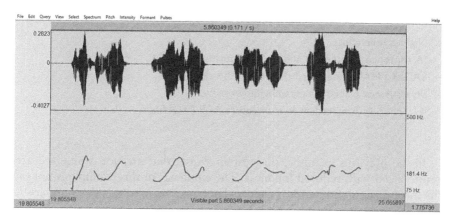

Figure 2.4 Melodic monotony, produced with the PRAAT software

regardless of the meaning of the sentences. If the listeners are aware of this speaking style, it can distract them from the message. The listener will not always be able to identify the nature of the abnormal speech pattern but will likely lose attention regardless, due to the speaking style sounding dull (monotony) or confusing (melodic monotony).

In addition to prosodic problems at the sentence level, problems can also occur at the word level. These are related to syllabic stress. For example, the word "irresistible" is pronounced /IRRESTIBLE/. Moreover, unstressed syllables are often omitted, as in the word "irresponsible" being pronounced /IRSPONSIBLE/. If such word structure errors occur frequently and regularly, they can distract the listener's attention from the content of the message. In an effort to avoid being boring, many speakers — not just the PWC — emphasize short words that are of less semantic importance at the beginning of their sentences. The following example demonstrates how the sentence emphasizes prepositions rather than meaningful words:

> At the campsite IN the small village, IN this case, a bad meal is given TO people.

Abnormal stress patterns

Due to the wrong stress pattern, the message in the statement "That HAP-PENS daily" can elude the listener. The accent in the example above was made with variations in loudness and pitch. The trailing of the volume at the end of a sentence (the so-called night candle effect) is a common phenomenon in cluttering (see the example below). The night candle effect negatively affects the speaker's intelligibility and the listener's ability to understand.

> Night candle effect
> (A sentence starts loud and ends in murmuring)
> SADLY I HAVE not heard the end of the sentence
> Stress is not placed on meaningfull words:
> IN a shop in Amsterdam four sweaters ARE STOLEN

In the previous example, the written words that are not capitalized are pronounced with reduced loudness. The emphasis in this example is not on the most meaningful words. Listeners later ask, "Where was this burglary?" and "Where were sweaters stolen?"

2.2.7   *Rhythm and musicality*

A disturbed speech rhythm combined with tachylalia (speech that is too fast) or bradylalia (speech that is too slow), is considered by many to be a good indicator of cluttering (Daly, 1996; St. Louis, 1992; St. Louis et al., 2003; van Zaalen et al., 2008). The speech intelligibility of PWC can be affected by surges of fast speech. Speech disorders become even more apparent when the surges of fast speech are combined with short pauses between sentences and rapid speech at the beginning of sentences. These abrupt beginnings sometimes lead to staccato speaking.

The problems become even more severe for PWC when they have to memorize or retell children's poems, because such poems are based mainly on repeated, rhythmic patterns. The reduced correlation between the rhythmic pattern and the pauses (phrasing) leads to serious phrasing problems, which further disrupt speech intelligibility. Treatment can be highly challenging if such problems are caused by a lack of musical (sensory) characteristics. These musical characteristics are not the same as musicality.

2.2.8 *Handwriting and writing problems*

Sufficient language skills (reading, speaking, writing, and listening) are essential for efficient, easy, and effective communication with others. It is well known that PWC may experience difficulties in any of the four language modalities. The difficulties occur when the rate does not match the speaker's abilities. If the rate of PWC is slower and their focus on speech is greater, the problems in language skills temporarily disappear.

Problems of the PWC in writing are examined by multiple researchers (Daly & Cantrell, 2006; Bezemer et al., 2010; Dinger et al., 2008; van Zaalen & Winkelman, 2009, 2014). Pilot research shows a strong correlation between different rates of movement such as in walking, speaking, and writing, or, as some mothers may say, "He walks fast, he talks fast, and he thinks fast."

Writing is learning how culturally specific characters are represented based on certain distinct shapes, relationships, and measures. Writing is correlated with speech production; it is just another way to express the same speech and language code. Verbal language production is the development of successive movement patterns of breathing, vocal cords, labial, lingual, and jaw muscles. Handwriting is a traceable form of movements that visualizes internal speech through sound symbols. Where a phonetic plan leads to a speech motor plan of spoken language, a phonetic plan leads to a grapheme-motor plan in written language. Readability depends on the shape, the movement track, and the space on the paper. The speed of writing is correlated with the speed of one's actions and thinking.

A child is already able to perform fine grapheme-motor movements at the age of three. Long before children enter kindergarten, they are already able to perform finger movements with eight millimeters of precision. These finger movements, used in writing and drawing, are therefore usually well-developed when children go to kindergarten. This does not mean that fine motor development is completed at that age. Writing is still an essential skill for adequate functioning in school.

> Lise, 9, claims: "When I pay attention to my writing, I do not know how to write the word anymore. Moreover, if I pay close attention to how the word should be written, I can no longer write neatly."

In recent years there has been more attention on learning to write, but the prevalence of writing problems is nevertheless increasing. In a study of children aged eight to thirteen years, Van Hoorn et al. (2010) found percentages of children with poor handwriting (2 percent with dysgraphia and 19 percent with poor handwriting). PWC often make spelling errors that are correlated with speech errors. The significant variation in the prevalence of dysgraphic handwriting (5 to 33 percents) is of clinical importance, because poor handwriting has been identified as one of the most common reasons for referring school-age children to occupational therapy or physical therapy, and it is included as a criterion for the diagnosis of developmental coordination disorder (Overvelde & Hulstijn, 2011). Among 4th-grade students, Rubin and Henderson (1982) found a lower percentage of children with "severe handwriting problems" (i.e., 12.3 percent) compared to students in lower grades. Maeland (1992) reported that 9.6 percent of "clumsy" ten-year-old children had "handwriting problems," while Karlsdottir and Stefansson (2002) classified 13 percent of 307 five-year-old elementary school children as students with dysfunctional handwriting. The researchers indicated that handwriting should not be assessed during group 2 but should be postponed to group 3 or later.

No scientific studies have been published on handwriting problems and cluttering, as far as we have been able to ascertain. However, our clinical experience indicates that writing problems in PWC are frequently evident. A person with syntactic cluttering produces a high frequency of word repetitions and revisions in both written and spoken language; a person with phonological cluttering presents with a higher-than-normal number of illegible words due to telescopic production of graphemes. PWC who want to write "beautifully" inhibit their high speed while writing, which leads to increased pressure on the paper they write so that they complain of fatigue while writing. If the writing is exhausting or unpleasant, these individuals will tend to write less and less.

2.2.9   *Self-assessment, speech control, and monitoring*

In the 1970s, many authors saw the sensory component as a causative and a maintaining factor of cluttering (St. Louis et al., 2007). According to these authors, the self-monitoring by PWC was reduced. This explanation is very plausible, given that PWC are usually unaware of their problems in fluency and speech intelligibility, which is consistent with the belief that the sensory component is a maintaining factor. The poor intelligibility of speech is caused by a specific deficit in language formulation, fast speech rate, abnormal timing, and irregular rhythm. But it is essential to emphasize that when the language formulation component is not a problem, PWC are fully capable of self-monitoring their speech. Therefore, the sensory component is ruled out as the primary cause of cluttering.

2.2.10.   *Attention and focus*

Kussmaul noted in 1877 that more focused attention improves speech production in PWC. Conversely, cases of less focused attention clearly expose more cluttering symptoms. Many parents or other relatives of PWC have confirmed these observations over the years.

> Romy, who is married to a person with cluttering, remarked, "Lately, Kawin has been completely unintelligible when he talks to me. But, when he talks to my friends, he is suddenly intelligible. Sometimes it feels like he doesn't want to do his best for me anymore."

The speech production of PWC usually deteriorates during relaxation; however, their speech usually improves when they participate in a conversation with unfamiliar people. The reason for this speech improvement is that PWC become more focused and alert due to the presence of unfamiliar people. This aspect of cluttering may mislead the referring physician or speech therapists during the diagnostic evaluation. Often people feel uncomfortable during their first sessions with the therapist. They experience problems with speech but want to show what they are capable of. As a result, they turn their attention to their speech and show fewer symptoms than they usually would. In later sessions, when clients experience less tension, they will be less alert, and their cluttering will increase. To detect speech errors during the first sessions, the Predictive Cluttering Inventory-revised (PCI-r) (See Section 1.4.5 and Appendix A) and the Screening Phonological Accuracy (Appendix E) may be used. In addition, speech can be assessed in less structured circumstances, where PWC are unaware that their speech is being recorded.

2.2.11 Auditory skills

The correlation between cluttering and possibly impaired auditory processing skills has recently attracted more interest among researchers than in prior years. One of the explanations is the temporary positive effect of auditory feedback through headphones, by using heightened auditory feedback (HAF) or delayed auditory feedback (DAF). auditory feedback or delayed auditory feedback, DAF). This can be explained by the 40-second rule. When examining the reading skills of children with cluttering, DAF can reduce cases of word omissions, guesses in reading, and phonological paraphasias. However, although not expected it is not clear whether PWC have abnormal auditory memory, or problems in auditory analysis, synthesis, discrimination, or processing. PWC make mistakes when verbally repeating sentences, which causes them to have a low score on auditory memory tasks. However, when PWC are asked to write down sentences, they generally do not make mistakes or leave anything out, so the problem seems to lie in production and not in memory.

Errors in auditory memory tasks

In all likelihood, the mistakes made in reciting sentences are mainly caused by a speed that is inappropriate for the task. When repeating these sentences while wearing headphones, PWC no longer make the abovementioned errors.

Given that PWC generally have no difficulties focusing their attention, any problems they may experience in auditory skills can be considered an additional problem or a correlated problem.

2.2.12   Planning problems

Many speech therapists are familiar with the phenomenon that PWC often have difficulty being on time for therapy, as in the following example.

Wednesday at 8:45 A.M., Martin has an appointment at the dentist. It is a ten-minute bike ride from his house to the dentist. At 8:35 A.M., Martin decides he wants to take a shower. After all, a shower only lasts five minutes. Later, he is shocked that he is late for his dentist appointment once again!

Clearly, Martin thinks about the time he needs for the actions that need to be carried out. However, at the same time, he pays no attention to the time needed for showering and cycling, not to mention the time required to dress and undress, walk to the bike, grab, and lock the bike again, and walk from the parked bike to the dental office.

We assume that PWC experience planning problems in their speech, writing, and daily general and financial activities. Unfortunately, although interesting, there is no research data available on this topic. Therefore, a conclusion on the presence of planning problems for PWC will not be drawn now.

2.3   Influences on speech rate

Figure 2.5 shows the external influences on the rate of speech. These influences are discussed in detail in the following paragraphs. Finally, the mean articulatory rate in syllables per second is shown in Chapter 1, Figure 1.4

2.3.1   Linguistic factors

Several linguistic/linguistic factors influence speech and articulatory rates. It is well known that syllables within the first words of utterances are produced

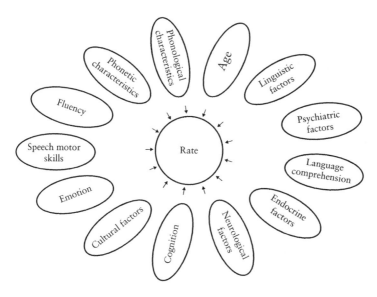

Figure 2.5 External influences on the speech rate

faster than the same syllables at the end of utterances. The complexity of the sentence also affects the speech rate; the more complex the sentence structure, the more interjections and pauses take place, which slows down the speech rate. In addition, several researchers have found that longer sentences are produced slightly faster than shorter ones (for example, Kelly & Conture, 1992). The speech rate is influenced by the conversational interaction rate, also referred to as the speed of turn-taking or the interaction rate, also known as the speed of the turn taking. During a conversation where the normal pause duration of 0.5–1.0 seconds is reduced, the speech rate of the following utterance will be faster than in a dialogue where sufficiently long pauses are used.

2.3.2 *Phonetic and phonological aspects*

The duration of the syllable depends on the number of sounds per syllable, the stress pattern, and the word length. For example, the duration of a syllable composed of several consonants and a vowel, such as "spread," is significantly longer (mean 0.32 seconds) than that of a syllable consisting of two consonants and a vowel, such as "cook" (mean 0.19 seconds). A syllable also lasts longer when produced in the front of the mouth, such as "pip" (mean 0.22 seconds), compared to when it is produced in the back of the mouth, such as "kick" (mean 0.19 seconds). In addition to the pitch adjustment, the stress on a syllable is also made by adjusting the duration of a syllable. Syllables within a long multisyllabic word are generally spoken faster than syllables within a short word.

2.3.3   *Relevance of the topic to the speaker*

The speech rate is highly dependent on the topic's relevance to the speaker. When speakers are asked to give their opinion, the rate at which this will be implemented will depend heavily on the theme's relevance. For example, a student member of the school board will give her opinion on the number of contact hours at a higher rate than a student who is not a member of the board. The number of times an opinion is formulated also influences the speech rate. The more often people tell the same story, the more their speech rate will increase. It is essential for speech therapists to properly understand any differences in rate and/or comprehensibility and intelligibility. Analyzing speech-language production at different levels of language complexity and whether the client is aware or not aware of the recording is of paramount importance (See Chapter 7, Section 7.2).

2.3.4   *Influence of speech rate on perceptions of the speaker*

The speech rate may vary depending on the social context. A person with a slow speech rate is usually seen as "professional" or "confident," but a person with an excessively fast speech rate is usually considered "passionate" or "nervous." On the other hand, a person who speaks quickly without disfluencies can be seen as very confident or even overwhelming or dominant. Within families, unspoken comments are often implied. An expression like "He talks like a real Gillisen" exemplifies this. Self-image usually develops from the time of adolescence. Adolescence is the period in which the articulatory rate is highest (See Chapter 1, Section 1.4.8). Therefore, it is expected that people's self-image can influence their speech rate, especially during and after adolescence.

Notwithstanding the above, it cannot necessarily be concluded that slow speakers with a low pitch voice generally come across as confident. There is apparently also an intergenerational difference in perception of rate, as shown by Apple et al. (1979) experiments. In their study, 61 students listened to recordings of male speakers answering two interview questions and then rated the speakers on different semantic differential scales. The pitch of the speakers' voices could be increased or decreased by 20 percent (or left at the normal level), and the speech rate could be increased or reduced by 30 percent (or remain unchanged). The results provided clear evidence that listeners use these acoustic characteristics when making personal judgments about speakers. Speakers with high voices were rated as less truthful, emphatic, less convincing (smaller, weaker, faster), and more nervous. Slow speakers were found to be less truthful, less fluent, and less persuasive, and were seen as more "passive" but more "powerful." However, the effects of the acoustic manipulations on personal attributions also depended on the specific question that provoked the reaction. If the speaker tells a story many times, the speech rate will be higher than when first told. After all, the rate is not interfered with by the time it takes to retrieve words and formulate sentence constructions. This is, of course, limited by the individual level of speech motor skills and phonetic and phonological aspects of the message.

2.3.5 *Speech rate in people with intellectual or neurological disabilities*

Contrary to generally prevailing expectations, people with intellectual disabilities appear to have an articulatory and speech rate similar to controls (Coppens-Hofman et al., 2013). Coppens-Hofman et al. found that since the average articulatory rate of the adults in their study was comparable to that of adults without intellectual disabilities, there was no evidence that their speech rate was affected by their disability. The authors of this study did not find a significant correlation between the speech rate and the number or type of disfluencies. Thus, the idea that people with intellectual disabilities necessarily speak slowly was unsubstantiated and was probably based solely on the listeners' perceptions. The speech of people with intellectual disabilities can be perceived as slow based on the high frequency of typical disfluencies and the content of their messages related to their intellectual level. Changes in speech rate can be noted in people with some neurological disorders, especially those involving the basal ganglia or the language formulation areas. The speech rate may decrease or increase due to the above-mentioned conditions. Examples of disorders associated with a high speech rate are Parkinson's disease, Wernicke's aphasia, Fragile-X syndrome, ADHD/ADD, and manic episodes (See Chapter 5, Sections 5.1 and 5.2).

2.3.6 *Emotional condition and motivation*

The intrinsic motivation to share a message affects the speaker's speech rate. When speakers are not particularly interested in a topic, their speech rate will be much slower than when the same speakers cover topics they are passionate about. The endocrine system or hormone system is the organ system that is responsible for a person's hormonal balance. That hormone strongly influences the speech rate and can even make previously inaudible symptoms noticeable. This is very clear in preadolescence, where the articulatory rate increases under the influence of the hormone balance, which can initiate symptoms of cluttering. The hormonal balance stabilizes after adolescence. The endocrine system is also closely involved in human emotions. For example, extroversion, enthusiasm, and anger are also associated with a high speech rate, and the social attractiveness of a person increases if the speech rate is comparable (Kallinen & Ravaja, 2004).

2.3.7. *Effect of age*

There is a correlation between the speech rate of speakers and their age. Very young children and very old adults speak significantly slower than adolescents and young adults (Quené, 2011; van Zaalen & Winkelman, 2009). Varia-tions in speech rates may also be related to other differences, such as gen-der, education level, regional background, mean length of utterance, average lexical diversity (Quené, 2011), ethnicity, and life experiences. Quené (2011) found that older listeners' perceptions can be influenced by their own speech rate, due to age-related changes in their articulation and in their cognitive abilities. Quené hypothesized that the stimulus-speech rate that listeners con-sider to be the most comfortable is identical to their own speech rate.

2.3.8.   *Measurement of the rate in a person's first or second language*

A recent study by Nagy et al. (2020) compared two methods of calculat-ing the articulation rate automatically and explored whether the speech rate is a valid measure of proficiency when social factors and proficiency vary independently. The study resolved several difficulties when using articula-tion rate as a measurement for more labor-intensive proficiency processing of spontaneous speech data. The findings of Nagy et al. (2020) suggested that the speech rate was a valid measurement of heritage language proficiency. The factor with the most substantial effect is the generation after immigra-tion (indicating the dominant language in the speaker's community during childhood years). The effects of social influences are complicated but must be explored to interpret the proficiency measure correctly. The data of Bradlow (2019) revealed that the slow rate of L2 relative to L1 speech was due to temporal restructuring that went beyond an increase in segment, syl-lable, and word durations and that the resulting information rate of L2 speech deviates considerably from that of L1 speech. To our knowledge, multilingual research has not been done on the rate of PWC. We, therefore, recommend that, during the evaluation of cluttering, speech therapists should determine and interpret the speech rate in all languages spoken by the speaker.

2.4.   Conclusion

In this chapter, a wide range of symptoms related to cluttering were pre-sented. The type of symptoms and the frequency and extent to which symp-toms occur do not determine the severity of the condition. The severity of cluttering is ascertained by the extent to which PWC can adjust their speech rate to the linguistic and motor demands of the moment. Knowledge and understanding of the symptoms of cluttering can assist in assessing PWC and can also be used to explain to clients why their communication is disrupted.

Part 2

Diagnostics

3 Assessment

The diagnosis of cluttering depends on whether PWC manifest cluttering in a relatively pure form or whether cluttering is combined with other conditions, such as neurofibromatosis type 1 (NF1), ADHD/ADD, or stuttering. In the latter case, it is essential to recognize that cluttering sometimes does not emerge as a salient condition until the stuttering has subsided, either spontaneously or because of treatment, or at least during the process of treatment for stuttering. It is also important to document the possible presence of other coexisting difficulties with communication or learning (Van Zaalen et al., 2008).

Various tools to diagnose cluttering are available in multiple languages and are always focused on a diagnostic protocol. Cluttering is a syndrome with a wide variety of symptoms that only in combination can lead to a cluttering diagnosis. Some diagnostic tools distinguish certain aspects of cluttering from stuttering or other learning or communication disorders. The Fluency Assessment Battery (Van Zaalen & Reichel, 2015; Van Zaalen & Winkelman, 2009; Van Zaalen et al., 2011), renamed in 2022 as the Cluttering Assessment Battery (CAB), has been developed to analyze the speech behavior of people with problems in understanding, problems being understood, and/or fluency problems, as well as difficulties in all aspects of communication and speech production. The different components of the CAB are discussed in Chapter 4. Experts such as Scaler Scott (2020) and Neumann (2019) have endorsed the CAB. The CAB has been translated into many languages, including English, Dutch, Swedish, Norwegian, German, French, Arabic, Polish, Bulgarian, Portuguese, Italian, Spanish, Finnish, Chinese, Indonesian, Nigerian, Russian, and Lithuanian.

We want to stress that, according to the International Classification of Functioning, Disability and Health (ICF), an assessment should not focus solely on the limitations of PWC but should also emphasize the potential of PWC for change and development. The focus of the assessment should be on functioning and participation as well as recognition of the importance of personal and environmental factors. An important goal in the diagnostic phase is to investigate the different processes of language production in relation to

DOI: 10.4324/9781003460558-5

each other, distinguishing them from other speech, language, and fluency disorders. Another important objective is to consider or exclude other disorders, such as learning disabilities, dyslexia, ADHD/ADD, Down syndrome, fragile X syndrome, NF1, or intellectual disabilities. Because cluttering can mask all the above issues, the CAB has been developed so that data collected in this assessment tool can be easily applied to other diagnostic tools, such as the Stuttering Severity Instrument (Riley, 2009).

3.1   Predictive Cluttering Inventory-revised

In 2006, Daly and Cantrell presented their latest checklist of symptoms, which they called the Predictive Cluttering Inventory (PCI). This checklist is based on the opinions of international experts regarding symptoms related to cluttering. The PCI contains 33 items that are clinically observed in different PWC. A later study found that the 2006 version of the PCI needed to be standardized in order to be specific and sensitive enough to detect possible cluttering (Van Zaalen et al., 2009c). Based on the item analysis, only ten items in the 2006 version of the PCI were found to show significant differences between cluttering and other conditions. These items are utilized in the revised PCI, a standardized checklist for cluttering-like speech (See Chapter 1, Section 1.4.5). Although these items are not always 100 percent clear, this updated checklist can help speech therapists detect symptoms and determine whether further evaluation is necessary using the CAB. The PCI-revised version also gives speech therapists a clear understanding of the linguistic and communicative characteristics of the PWC. The instruction and interpretation are described in Chapter 1, Section 1.4.5.

3.2   History taking

The differential diagnosis between cluttering and coexisting disorders, such as specific language impairment (SLI), learning difficulties, or ADHD/ADD, is not easy to arrive at for children until they reach the age of ten. Because language development is never finished, the diagnosis of cluttering is not always definite. For more information on the differential diagnosis between various fluency disorders, see Chapter 5. As with most speech-language evaluations, the history taking should include information on the following five aspects:

1 Complaints and expectations of PWC.
2 Birth and developmental history.
3 Medical history.
4 Timeline and effectiveness of previous treatment.
5 Family history of speech or language disorders, including attention problems, fluency disorders and tachylalia.

1 Complaints and expectations of PWC

When taking a history, the speech therapist must find out why PWC signed up for an assessment (and possible treatment) at this point in their lives. The reason for seeking assessment and treatment strongly impacts the intervention goals and the internal motivation of PWC to change. Complaints of PWC can result from tension within the communication context or negative external feedback to their speech.

The question of whether clients understand the impact of their speech production compared to their actual difficulty or external complaints of listeners should be raised. Answers to these questions will provide speech therapists with an idea of the extent to which PWC understand the deficits underlying their communication problems. Before the speech therapist starts an intervention, PWC should be asked which situations they consider the most important for changing their speech. Cluttering is not easy to treat, and full recovery is not certain. The therapy will benefit significantly if the treatment goals reflect the expectations and needs of the client.

2 Birth and developmental history

While no genetic factors have been identified for cluttering, gathering a birth history will assist speech therapists in better understanding the cluttering disorder, and will provide other important information about the causes of this condition. Information about developmental history is important because it describes indicators of cluttering that may influence the client's perception of their own behavior. In addition to an assessment of speech and language, developmental history can suggest other potential treatment goals. Handwriting problems, for example, are not recognized as related to the spoken messages in many adults with cluttering who begin therapy; they feel like this is a separate disorder. Difficulty with handwriting can be part of the same compromised speech and language production system. In our experience, adults with cluttering are relieved to discover that some of their symptoms are part of the same underlying deficiency and that they are not related to different disorders.

> The client, Sanne, expressed her relief as follows: "Oh, sometimes I just started doubting myself, because I make mistakes in so many things. I'm so glad I now know that my effort to slow down can cause things to go wrong on multiple fronts."

It is also helpful to study the history of potentially relevant symptoms, regardless of whether they have led to formal diagnoses, such as behavioral problems or ADHD/ADD, learning disabilities, and an auditory processing disorder in school or work environments. These additional problems can have severe implications for the assessment and therapy planning of the

PWC (See Chapter 6). Additional information on differential diagnostics will be provided later in this chapter.

3   Medical history

Medical history information is important for two reasons. First, this information may affect treatment planning and/or treatment outcomes; and second, gathering information about the PWC as a group may help researchers in the future. An important aspect of medical history is whether a client is taking medications that may affect their attention or speech rate.

Various medications, such as Levodopa, Ritalin, and antidepressants, are known for their influence on speech and language fluency. Little is known about the effects of other drugs on speech rates and control. Research regarding the effects of medications on cluttering has not been conducted to date, possibly because pharmaceutical companies do not see disorders such as cluttering to be economically attractive to their profit margins. Suppose a client uses medications that may affect attention, language formulation, or speech production. In such cases, speech therapists should consult their client's physicians to determine whether adjusting the dosage of the medications might be beneficial to the success of the client's speech therapy.

4   Timeline and effectiveness of previous treatment

The date of the initial treatment can give speech therapists a clear idea of the time in the client's speech development when the first critical symptoms emerged to lead to seeking a speech and language evaluation. For example, clients who begin therapy to improve rate-related symptoms are more likely to improve if they begin therapy during adolescence than if they begin therapy in early childhood (See Figure 3.1).

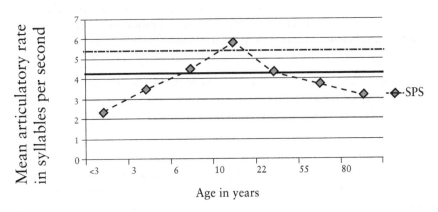

Figure 3.1 Correlation between mean articulatory rate (in syllables per second) and language production

Figure 3.1 shows an example of the effect of dissociation between rate and language formulation: The solid unbroken line indicates the maximum rate at which client A can speak fluently or intelligibly. In the case of client A, cluttering symptoms will be apparent from age seven to eight, and will not really change during this client's childhood and early adulthood. Client B (starred line) is disfluent or unintelligible at a rate of 5.3 syllables per second (SPS). Client B will experience cluttering symptoms in early adolescence (when the speech rate reaches 5.4 SPS) and is likely to recover in early adulthood, when the rate will naturally decline. Client C speaks at a normal rate and is represented by the broken line consisting of dashes and squares.

Clients looking for cluttering therapy often have some experience with previous therapy, which they indicate has not been beneficial. One of the explanations for this hop-on hop-off approach to therapy is the clients' inconsistent desire to control their speech rate: They are eager to change their speech rate but sometimes lack the intrinsic motivation to continue to monitor/inhibit their fast rate of speech. Another explanation can be found in treating only some of the symptoms associated with cluttering, such as improvement of language abilities or merely by working on producing specific sounds.

Effective and evidence-based therapy methods, such as audio-visual feedback training (see Chapter 7, Section 7.4), have a good chance of being effective again later in life. Although there is no guarantee that the method will work with a second round of therapy, using different treatment methods at the beginning of therapy is unnecessary. This is especially true when speech therapists follow the client's ideas about effective treatment. In addition, if the client is convinced that a method has been or will be effective, their internal motivation will be strengthened.

5 Family history of speech or language disorders, including attention problems, fluency disorders, and tachylalia

Several researchers have concluded that there is a high probability that family members of PWC have a speech or language disorder. Information on the occurrence of attention problems, hyperactivity, fluency disorders, dyslexia, and tachylalia in family members is very important due to group dynamics. For example, it is very difficult for one person in a family of fast speakers to slow down when everyone else is speaking very fast.

> Change the speech behavior within the whole family, not just the person with cluttering. For example, when you think of a car, can you imagine trying to slow down only one of the wheels? Obviously not! All four wheels need to be slowed down.

If cluttering or tachylalia occurs in the family, it is advisable to work with all family members simultaneously, if they are available. The main goal for the family will be an appropriate change in their behavior. There is no need to formally "treat" all family members. All assessment procedures are detailed in Part 2, "Diagnostics."

3.3   Considerations around bilingualism and cluttering

In Chapter 2, Section 2.3.7, the speech rate in relation to bilingualism is discussed. More research needs to be conducted on cluttering and multi-lingualism. Dalton and Hardcastle (1993) pointed out that their bilingual clients from Pakistan and India exhibit some rhythmic non-cluttering patterns in their first language. Dalton and Hardcastle, therefore, propose to re-examine the first languages of PWC in order to adapt treatment strategies to the specific problems of their clients. They also recommend assessing the relationship between the types of disfluencies presented by speakers of different languages and the characteristics of those languages, such as rhythm and articulation patterns. It is worth repeating that these proposals are based on clinical observation, not empirical evidence. Switching between languages is a strenuous cognitive retrieval process. These increased demands can cause changes in the symptoms of bilingual speakers with cluttering (Hernandez, 2009).

When a bilingual person speaks their second language fluently and quickly enough, cluttering symptoms may surface. If the speaker does not have a sufficient command of the second language, the search for words and sentence constructions will slow the speech rate to such an extent that cluttering symptoms will be minimal.

3.4   Audio- and video-recordings

To analyze cases of cluttering, assessment procedures should include examples of spontaneous speech and dialogue (with a duration of three to ten minutes), perhaps in unconventional environments (for example, when speakers do not know they are being recorded, subject to the procedure described below), and at different levels of language complexity. In addition, digital video and audio recordings are recommended for analyses of fluency, rate and rate adjustment, sentence and word structure, and intelligibility in various speaking tasks for people with possible cluttering.

Speech therapists should know that when recorded, PWC will try to "normalize" speech behavior. Therefore, speech therapists can prevent possible bias by comparing the communication behavior of PWC when they are aware of the recording with those when they speak spontaneously and are unaware of the recording.

As noted earlier, a person with cluttering can monitor their speech for an average of 30 to 40 seconds (40-second rule). While recording the client, the speech therapist needs to repeatedly interrupt the client, knowing that after each interruption, the client will be able to monitor their speech for this period of time. Therefore, the recording of the client's spontaneous speech needs to start 40 seconds after each interruption.

Note: It is considered unethical to record a client's speech without revealing that these recordings are being made. At the speech therapist's first face-to-face meeting with the client and their parent(s) or partner, the speech therapist must ask for permission to make audio and/or video recordings. Once a consent form is signed, family members can record the client's speech behavior when the client is unaware of it. Usually, this is done at home, with a laptop or a mobile phone. As long as the client has given prior permission, these recordings can be shared with and saved by the speech therapist.

The differential diagnosis performed during the CAB administration should be recorded via audio and video. The CAB consists of various tasks, including oral reading, spontaneous speech, retelling a memorized story, writing, screening for phonological accuracy, a test of oral-motor coordination, and questionnaires. Additional receptive and expressive language tests can serve as diagnostic tools to rule out a language disorder.

Cluttering is more likely to emerge when the speaking task is more spontaneous and informal, less structured, more emotionally and linguistically complex, or when the client should be made aware that she is being recorded. The severity of cluttering can vary depending on the nature of the speaking task and is determined by the level of language complexity when the symptoms are audible. The lower the language complexity in which symptoms occur, the more severe the cluttering is. We have encountered many PWC whose cluttering could be identified only at the highest levels of language complexity. However, the severity of cluttering is not only determined by the level of language complexity in which it occurs but also by the impact it has on the person's social functioning.

> Mohammed can control his speech well at most levels of language complexity, but if he wants to convince others of something, he loses his speech control. During arguments, he speaks with so many typical disfluencies that the listeners are hardly open to the content of his arguments. Convincing Mohammed's brother Steven would not be a problem for him. Mohammed works as a salesperson in an antique shop. He needs help to persuade skeptical patrons to buy their items. His boss, who referred him for therapy, has linked Mohammed's therapy success to his job retention.

3.5 Speech rate adjustment

PWC cannot adjust their speech rate to the linguistic (syntactic or phonological) demands of the moment. In a linguistically challenging context, people usually speak more slowly; they adjust their speech rate to retrieval time to select words and formulate the ideas that they want to express. People generally speak faster when they talk about simple things or tell the same stories for the third or fourth time. The reason for a lower rate in more difficult speech conditions is apparent: utterances used frequently have a shorter retrieval time than utterances used for the first time. Typical speakers use a slower rate when communicating in a second or third language. This is certainly the case if the second or third language is not sufficiently mastered. PWC show a need for adjustment of their rate to the linguistic demands of the moment. Their articulatory rate remains the same at different levels of language complexity. When performing a complex language task, their speech rate remains the same, even if retrieval or formulation of sentences takes much longer. Based on clinical experience and tens of thousands of measurements using PRAAT software, we have found that fluent people read aloud, retell a story, and speak spontaneously at different speech rates. These speech rate differences between speaking tasks range between 1.0 and 3.3 SPS, measured as a product of the highest and lowest mean articulatory rates produced.

In the cases of PWC, the adjustment of the mean articulatory rate between the three speech conditions just mentioned is less than 1.0 SPS.

Oliver speaks with an average articulatory rate of 5.4 SPS (spontaneous speech), 5.6 SPS (retelling), and 6.0 SPS (reading aloud). The variation between tasks is < 1.0 SPS. This is an indication of cluttering. If Oliver also presents with at least one of the core symptoms of cluttering, and there are no other explanations for these core symptoms, the diagnosis of cluttering is confirmed.

Another way to assess the capacity for rate adjustment is to ask PWC to speak or read faster. Fluent speakers and PWS will increase their articulatory rate, while PWC will engage in hasty or relaxed behavior without talking faster or slower.

Assessment of cluttering should be performed with tasks at different rates, at different levels of language complexity, and with and without a focus on speaking.

3.6 Fluency

If a speaker frequently presents with interjections and revisions, this has implications for the perception of abnormal fluency in PWC (Starkweather, 1987; Logan & LaSalle, 1999; see Section 2.2.4). It has been postulated that some of the disfluencies exhibited by PWC are caused by linguistic, rather than motor problems. These disfluencies are often called 'linguistic maze', (Howell & Au-Yeung, 2002), resulting in typical disfluencies (Van Zaalen et al., 2008); see also Section 1.5.3). According to Howell and Au-Yeung (2002), typical disfluencies are produced to gain time to plan the next linguistic structure. PWC typically say what is already planned.

The disfluency occurs when a person with cluttering tries to plan the remaining segment of a sentence. Once the next plan is prepared, the speech becomes fluent, and the remaining structure is executed as intended.

Therefore, disfluencies that are considered typical lack tension and are produced in normal rhythmic patterns. However, unlike stuttering-like disfluencies, typical disfluencies do not break up the syllable structure. The syllable remains intact. Typical disfluencies consist of one or two repetitions of syllables, words, and/or sentences, produced with a regular rhythm, without tension and additional stress. When assessing clients with fluency disorders, it is essential to examine the effect of language complexity on the type and frequency of disfluencies. The language formulation is influenced by the fast speech rate of PWC, depending on the level of language complexity. One way to test the correlation between the speech rate and language formulation is to ask PWC to communicate at different conversational levels, such as speaking spontaneously or retelling a story.

The speech therapist can then compare the effect of the linguistic task with the frequency and type of typical and stuttering-like disfluencies. A more complex task is ordinarily accompanied by an increased number of typical disfluencies and a slower rate.

The complexity level of the task should be high enough to trigger typical disfluencies and easy enough to allow the PWC to be successful without causing resistance. For a complete description of language complexity, see Chapter 7, Section 7.2.

3.7 Intelligibility

Impaired speech intelligibility is a core feature of a subtype of cluttering referred to as phonological cluttering (see also Chapter 1, Section 1.4.10). Intelligibility assessment should include tasks ranging from short and structured to longer and less structured. Examples of the first are rote tasks, such as counting or retelling a story. Speech therapists should be alert to errors in syllable- and word structure and should measure the articulatory rate. Some PWC tend to present phoneme-specific errors. Most PWC exhibit reduced non-phoneme-specific speech intelligibility as their language becomes more informal and their utterances become lengthier. Omissions of sounds and syllables, neutralization of vowels, and cluster reductions can affect speech intelligibility. Impaired speech intelligibility is often associated with limited jaw movement while talking, which also decreases resonance. This limited jaw movement automatically improves when the PWC speaks more slowly, such as when reading aloud.

Simple tests to assess intelligibility

- Ask the client to count from 20 to 29.
- Ask the client to count backward.
- Ask the client to count backward and skip two numbers each time, for example, 100–97–94–91 and so on.

Children with cluttering who are up to 10.8 years of age old should be asked to read some words that are difficult to pronounce (for example, "statistical," "chrysanthemum," "possibilities," and "tyrannosaurus"), and should be asked to produce these words three times consecutively, first at a comfortable articulatory rate and then at a faster rate. An advanced test to assess intelligibility and phonological encoding is entitled Screening Phonological Accuracy." (See Chapter 4, Section 4.6.6)

3.8   Awareness and lack of awareness

When PWC focus on speech production, their fluency, and intelligibility improve over a short period, usually for 30 to 40 seconds. PWC sometimes complain that when they initially seek professional help, speech therapists cannot detect speech disorders, so they are sent home without treatment. The focus of PWC on speech production can explain their "good" speech during the intake process. It is therefore wise for the speech therapist to pass judgment on the speech-language production of PWC only after recordings have been analyzed in which the PWC speak freely and may not be aware of the recording. Parents and other family members sometimes tell the speech therapist that their child is unwilling to pay enough attention to their speech. They conclude that unfocused speech production in the home situation is less fluent and less intelligible than it is when other people are around. The speech therapist's assessment should be based on recordings of focused speech, i.e., times when the PWC are aware that they are being recorded, and of unfocused speech, times when the PWC are unaware that they are being recorded. Differences between these two sets of conditions provide essential information to the speech therapist regarding the clients' potential to change. Again, the clients must authorize the recording (See Section 3.4).

3.9   Linguistic skills

PWC often experience language problems in addition to their speech problems.

Problem or disorder?

In this instance, the word "problem" is deliberately chosen instead of "disorder." In principle, the speech and language production of PWC are well developed. However, at the fast rate of communication, PWC are unable to adjust their articulatory rate to linguistic demands, resulting in reduced intelligibility and comprehensibility. When the rate is slowed down, PWC do not experience these problems.

Language problems in PWC consist of word-finding difficulties, poor syntactic structure, lack of coherence in discourse and stories, and compromised pragmatics (for example, abnormal presuppositions, such as not considering the listener's point of view or knowledge, or frequent interruptions of an interlocutor's turn). However, with cluttering, most language problems disappear in linguistic contexts that are not complex. Many language problems in spoken language do not necessarily appear in written language. Language problems in cluttering, therefore, have to do with the rate of speech production and not with language disorders (Also see Chapter 1, Section 1.5.3, where cluttering is explained from a language automation model perspective).

This being said, it is necessary to assess the language skills of PWC. Language tests should be administered to rule out the possibility of additional language deficits as reasons for abnormal fluency. If PWC have receptive or expressive language deficits in addition to cluttering-like symptoms, a communication disorder should be considered and treated as a dual diagnosis in individuals with cluttering.

3.10   Oral-motor coordination

The diadochokinetic tasks of the Oral Motor Assessment Scale (OMAS) (Riley & Riley, 1985) provide clear guidelines for observation of oral-motor coordination skills. The oral-motor assessment provides information about the client's ability to coordinate muscle movements in repeated sequences of syllables, the productions of which require no linguistic competence. Therefore, no lexical retrieval and only limited phonological encoding are required during oral-motor assessment.

> In diadochokinetic tasks, the speech therapist assesses the ability to stop a specific motor impulse and replace it with an opposite movement. The relative timing is also called alternative motion rate (AMR) or sequential motion rate (SMR) (Juste et al., 2012).

The OMAS was standardized at a time when digital recordings were not available. Therefore, the OMAS was not standardized for adolescents or adults. In the revised version of OMAS by Van Zaalen and Winkelman (2009), the norms are available for all age groups, and are based on digital speech analysis performed using the speech analysis software Praat (Boersma & Weenink, 2022). Motor execution problems are not a symptom of cluttering. The OMAS is, therefore, administered to rule out the presence of motor execution problems that may be responsible for poor intelligibility. Someone who presents with difficulties on the OMAS and exhibits one or more symptoms of cluttering should be treated for cluttering as a second independent diagnosis.

3.11   Summary

Cluttering is a communication disorder in which people cannot adjust their speech rate to the linguistic and motor demands of the moment. This chapter has described the core characteristics and symptoms of cluttering. The fact that a fast speech rate affects both the speaker and the listener has been extensively discussed. Internal and external factors may also influence the client's speech or articulatory rate. To assess whether a person has a cluttering diagnosis, a thorough evaluation is necessary. The PCI-r is a good screening tool for identifying the possibility of cluttering. A comprehensive evaluation of cluttering, including taking a client's detailed history as well as presenting the CAB, will be discussed in Chapter 4.

4 Assessment instruments

4.1 The Cluttering Assessment Battery

The Cluttering Assessment Battery (CAB), see Appendices for the assessment forms, (Van Zaalen & Reichel, 2014; Van Zaalen & Winkelman, 2009) includes an analysis of the rate, fluency, intelligibility, and structure in various speech tasks: Spontaneous speech (see 4.6.2), reading aloud (see 4.6.3), retelling a story (see 4.6.4), writing and handwriting (see 4.6.5), the Screening Phonological Accuracy (SPA) (see 4.6.6), the Oral Motor Assessment Scale (OMAS) (see 4.6.7) and the Brief Stuttering and Cluttering Questionnaire (BSCQ) (see 4.6.8). Because many of the assessment tools used are language-specific, the assessment forms of the CAB are currently available in Dutch, Japanese, English, Finnish, French, Norwegian, Latvian, German, Italian, Lithuanian, and Polish. Translations into other languages will be forthcoming. In the diagnostic phase, therapy is begun by offering work-from-home exercises and evaluating them with the client.

When assessing cluttering, speech therapists investigate whether clients can adjust their speech rate to the linguistic demands of the moment. Speech therapists, therefore, compare the client's rate with their own speech rate. Comparison with population standards is not the primary goal for assessment. However, it is essential to evaluate to what extent the client's ability to focus and utilize auditory feedback influences the message delivery (comprehensibility) and intelligibility, regardless of whether the rate is adjusted or not.

4.2 Concomitant diagnostics and therapy

Therapy starts during the diagnostic phase. All speaking tasks are recorded and analyzed in the presence of the PWC. In this way, the PWC already gain insight into their own speaking behavior during the diagnostic process. This identification of symptoms is the first step in recognizing cluttering.

Diagnostic therapy, as described in Section 4.3, initiates the identification phase of cluttering therapy, and assesses the readiness of PWC to change their speaking behavior. In the identification phase, diagnostic therapy data

DOI: 10.4324/9781003460558-6

is collected, and based on this data, a treatment plan is mapped out. Since PWC are often unaware of their symptoms, it is especially important during the identification phase that PWC become aware of their symptoms and the problems they experience in communication. During this process, speech therapists gain insight into how much their clients can be stimulated. The defining question is: "Are their clients ready for change?" To be able to answer this question accurately, exercises are offered in the early identification phase. It is best to keep in mind that the exercises presented in the diagnostic therapy phase only provide information about the potential for change of the PWC and are not intended to be given as homework for more than one or two weeks. The exercises clarify the situation but will not lead to behavioral change.

A diagnosis can be made based on the information obtained in the diagnostic phase. This chapter describes the different aspects of the treatment plan. First, early transfer and stabilization is discussed, followed by some diagnostic exercises.

4.3   Diagnostic therapy (assessment and exercise)

The schedule of the first sessions varies with different PWC. Table 4.1 provides an example plan for the first four treatment sessions. As indicated in Chapter 1, internal monitoring, also referred to as feedback loop, of PWC is weak. Therefore, strengthening the feedback loop and assessing change readiness should be the primary goals during diagnostic therapy. As for the feedback loop, Levelt (1989) recommends three levels of monitoring (See Chapter 1, Section 1.6). The focus of PWC is on the third level. If the monitoring skills improve at this level of the language production process, they can work at the other two levels. As for the change in readiness, we refer to this in Section 4.4.

The weak monitoring skills of PWC are not necessarily clearly based on Levelt's model. It is well known that PWC do not sufficiently show symptom awareness (See the example below).

A therapist records her conversation with a client. She then plays it back. The client exclaims, "Wow, how did you do that!?" Only after multiple reactions by a client in this manner does the speech therapist realize that the client thinks that during the playback of the recording, the therapist left her own speech unchanged while changing the speech of the client to a fast, disfluent, and/or unintelligible speaking pattern. After this realization, it often takes the speech therapist more than one series of recordings to convince the client that what the client hears is entirely her own speech: unchanged but very fast, disfluent, and/or difficult to understand.

Table 4.1 Example of the planning for the first diagnostics and sessions (Van Zaalen & Winkelman, 2014)

Session (60 minutes) and goal	Procedures	Activity	Work at home
Session 1: Case history, start the Cluttering Assessment Battery	• Assess spontaneous speech, reading and SPA. • Determine the articulatory rate and ratio disfluencies (4.5.1 and 4.5.2). • Share information about cluttering.	• Tell me your name (4.3.1). • Read aloud a reading text adapted to the PWC level (Appendix L).	• Tell me your name (4.3.1). • Observe how often the PWC is asked, "What do you say?"
Session 2: Evaluation of Session 1 and the work-from-home assignment	• Perform other subtests of the Cluttering Assessment Battery: storytelling, OMAS, Speech Situation Checklist.	• Evaluate session 1 + home exercise • Recognize and describe difficult speaking situations.	• Collect multisyllabic words related to the profession or hobby of the PWC. • Speak for five minutes while tapping syllables. • Read aloud for five minutes daily. • Counting back one series daily. • Then, draw up a hierarchy of speaking situations.
Session 3: Evaluation of session two and work-from-home assignments	• Repeat the assessment components and interpret the level of language complexity in relation to the symptoms.	• Evaluate session 2 + home exercise • Start with the identification phase (See Part 3, "Therapy").	
Session 4: Evaluate the diagnostic process	• Repeat the assessment components on higher levels of language complexity and interpret the level of language complexity in relation to the symptoms. • Diagnosis	• Extensive evaluation • Start with the identification phase (See part 3, "Therapy").	

When working on monitoring, it is important to focus the attention of clients on identification, self-observation, and "speech awareness." The following exercises illustrate how to work on monitoring skills.

4.3.1 Diagnostic exercise 1 – Tell me your name

An excellent way to make PWC aware of their symptoms at the beginning of therapy is to give them a command, as described in this example.

The speech therapist asks the client: "This week when answering the phone, try to pronounce your name intelligibly." The difficulty the client experiences in pronouncing her name correctly increases her symptom awareness, and also the awareness of her own ability to start the process of change, which is referred to as the internal locus of control. Because pronouncing one's own name is more "personal" than any other word, it is sometimes necessary for the client to practice pronouncing their name during the session. If desired by the client and the therapist, this can be recorded and listened back to.

Experience shows that the voicemail messages of PWC are often less clear and fluent than those of speakers without speech problems. However, recording a correct voicemail message on other people's phones can be used (Winkelman, 1990).

Example of the exercise "Tell me your name."

Michael McKenzie (fictitious name) has been calling himself "Myksie" all his life. It is a big challenge for him to say his first and last name, producing five syllables instead of two. When the speech therapist pronounces Michael's full name in five syllables, he replies, "Yes, but I never say my name like that! It sounds weird." The speech therapist explains the purpose and subject of "adaptation." After saying his full name in five syllables five times in a row while tapping, Michael leaves the room feeling like he can change and is motivated to do the exercise daily.

The exercises in session 1, which involve pronouncing one's own name, may take time. Many speech therapists question whether the diagnostic assessment should be completed before giving home assignments or exercises. In cases of cluttering, this is certainly not true. Svend Smith, who also used his Accent method specifically for cluttering (Thyme-Frøkjær & Frøkjær-Jensen, 2004), practiced the principle that "during treatment the diagnosis becomes clear." In other words, the remaining steps in the assessment can be postponed until later in the program, and reevaluation during the treatment process is always beneficial. This reevaluation can potentially reveal several symptoms that were barely visible during the initial assessment. PWC find practicing and experiencing moments of success for the first time highly motivating. A therapist cannot start early enough.

4.3.2   Diagnostic exercise 2 – Articulatory rate

PWC must adjust their articulatory rate. In most cases, this means reducing the rate by syllable tapping or extending the pause duration. With syllable tapping, ask the client to pronounce each syllable clearly. This is not the same as "syllable tapping," as described in Chapter 7, Section 7.8. Understanding the client's ability to learn to adjust their articulatory rate is important. During the diagnostic phase, hard-to-pronounce multisyllabic words, such as those used in the SPA, can be practiced (see Chapter 4, Section 4.6.6). We prefer to use words related to the experience of the client, such as words related to their hobby or work. This increases their motivation to practice.

> In the first session, Anouk, 29, talked about her boyfriend's work as a "demi-logist." Writing down and producing the word "epidemiologist" was successful after the word was divided into syllables: /e/pi/de/mi/o/lo/gist/. After this, Anouk could produce the word correctly five times in a row. In the second session, she could pronounce her friend's profession correctly. This increased her sense of control and then motivated her to retrieve words that belonged to her repertoire and practice them.

Taking inventory of multisyllabic words in preparation for the syllable tapping assignment is an effective word-level exercise. In addition, it is advisable for PWC to practice producing multisyllabic words at different levels of complexity with different speaking rates. First, PWC should practice pronouncing words with three to five syllables. They should start with words they use every day, such as "hamburger," "computer," and "television." After this, the PWC may practice with more abstract words, such as "intelligence," "correspondence," and 'developmental care'. Such lists will help decide at which level of complexity to practice first. Generally, the rehearsed words should be "neither too easy nor too difficult." Accordingly, the PWC can be asked to write down multisyllabic words they hear, read, or use daily.

The level of complexity is related to phonology. For example, if the same sound appears in two consecutive syllables, one can be produced differently and with more effort due to the increased likelihood of coarticulation. Hence, the repeated production of the words "green gasses" is much more complex than the repeated production of the words "green grass." By repeating the words a few times in a row at a rapid rate, PWC are challenged to adjust their speech planning (during syllable tapping) to their sequential motor rate.

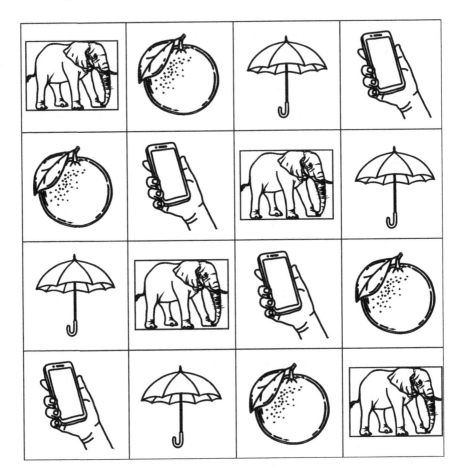

Figure 4.1 16 subjects – youth

For young children or individuals with dyslexia, working with images instead of written words is a good alternative. PWC may be asked to rapidly name objects within a field of 16 squares, in a specific order, based on the modeling of their speech therapist (see Figure 4.1). In Figure 4.1, the words "elephant," "telephone," "umbrella," and "mandarin" are produced as quickly as possible in different sequences (each row from left to right; each column from top to bottom; or zigzagging — first up, then down, and then up again, and so on). The goal is to remain intelligible and fluent. In addition, pauses between lines are not allowed.

Some children with cluttering find that when they speak quickly, they stumble over words, show hesitations, use fillers, repeat words, or need help to quickly retrieve words from their lexicon, effectively using time when they speak. One way to encourage children is to measure time with a stopwatch.

When shown the results, children are often surprised to find that when they speak slowly, they use less time than when they speak fast.

4.3.3 Diagnostic exercise 3 – Read aloud

Reading texts aloud, such as those used in the CAB, can serve as a diagnostic exercise with specific instructions (for example, reading rate). As long as it is a new text, it can improve symptom awareness. If improvement is noticed, the exercise can be used as a home assignment. However, the therapist should be aware that it is very important to select reading texts at the appropriate level — not too easy and not too challenging. The purpose of this exercise is not to make the client a better reader but to improve their speech mastery in circumstances that do not require language formulation skills (See also Chapter 7, Section 7.2.2).

Various exercises

Finding interesting reading texts can be quite challenging. An excellent alternative to routinely used exercises can be lyrics, especially from rappers, theater lyrics, and so forth. Such material can often be found on the Internet.

4.3.4 Diagnostic exercises 4 – Counting backward

Counting backward is much more difficult than reading aloud. This exercise was proposed by Kussmaul (1877) and Weiss (1964). As a diagnostic tool, this relatively challenging exercise can be applied appropriately to treating cluttering and stuttering. Counting backward can be used in the early stages of treatment in milder forms of cluttering. Winkelman (in Mensink-Ypma, 1990) didactically elaborated on the calculation exercises as follows:

Calculation exercises

Goal: Increase speech intelligibility at the word level.

How do you do it?

The client is asked to count aloud, subtracting two from 20 until the client reaches zero (20–18–16 till zero). Only the results are produced. A slightly more challenging variation is 100 minus two or five; 100 minus three or 300 minus seven are even more difficult. The arithmetic instruction should be difficult enough to increase focus and easy enough to pay sufficient attention to rate monitoring and speech production.

Possible effects

If the calculations are excessively challenging for the client, the breathing pattern may become dysrhythmic, and/or there may be an increase in typical disfluencies or especially /uh/ or /uhm/. If this happens, the speech therapist should give the client a more straightforward assignment, because when the client's attention decreases, word structure errors can occur. The risk increases after the first 30 to 40 seconds of the assignment.

Time investment

To get an idea of the duration of the assignment: 100 minus two to zero takes an average of 90 seconds; 100 minus three to one takes an average of 60 seconds.

(Winkelman, in Mensink-Ypma, 1990)

Utilizing math in the diagnostic phase of a person's therapy with cluttering has an important advantage over reading a text or retelling a story. When doing math exercises, linguistic requirements are lower, but mental activity is still necessary. By doing these exercises, the client's monitoring skills can also be improved. Another advantage of doing math exercises is that emotions rarely play a role when counting backward. An exception to this is during therapy with a very impatient client. With such clients, speech therapists may find themselves hitting a sore spot. Therefore, it is important to discuss the client's impatience or discomfort with math exercises. When the backward math exercise is adjusted to the client's level, this exercise can provide a good understanding of the client's ability to learn and make efforts after approximately a week.

Table 4.2 lists the types of attention and concentration in different speaking conditions.

Table 4.2 Types of attention and concentration during different speech conditions (Winkelman, 2006)

	Thinking	Language formulation	Emotions
Reading	–	–	–
Counting backward	+	–	–
Dialogue	+	+	+

4.4 Change readiness

Before the therapy can start, a therapist needs to know whether the PWC are ready for change; this is referred to as 'change readiness'. Determining the willingness to change is important for all clients, but certainly, for those who have cluttering. After all, the PWC themselves hardly suffer from speaking problems; the difficulty is experienced due to the listener's difficulties in understanding the speech of PWC. PWC have to work hard so that listeners can understand them. The question the therapist needs to ask is whether the PWC are ready for change. What is the motivation of the PWC? Table 4.3 details several considerations a therapist can make with PWC to determine if and when the PWC are open to change.

After the evaluation is completed, a comprehensive and individualized intervention plan can be developed. Sometimes PWC are unable to implement diagnostic exercises in their daily routine, despite the repeated instructions of their speech therapist. This could be an indication of resistance, which should be discussed between the speech therapist and the client. Such a scenario may be related to scheduling exercises over the course of the day. It is possible that simple tools, such as reminders on a computer or an alarm function on a mobile phone, can help the client plan and implement training schedules. However, in addition to finding the appropriate time slot to set aside for practice, there are many reasons why the intervention with the client may or may not be successful. These can include the people, the processes, the technological support and skills, the physical opportunities, and the organizational skills. We want to emphasize that both speech therapists

Table 4.3 Factors and considerations of readiness for change

Factors	Elements
At each stage of the therapy plan, consider the abilities of the speech therapist and the client to implement, integrate, and experience benefits from the therapy.	
People	Speech therapy experts, family, partners, friends, colleagues
	Knowledge/skills/abilities, experience, availability
Processes	Decision-making, therapy program management, strategy development, SMART goals
	Consistent practice with family
Technology support and skills	Software/hardware
	Habituation, familiarity, experience
Physical opportunities	Finances, space, and equipment (headphones, laptop)
	Expertise, availability
Organizational systems	Rewards, responsibility, exchange of knowledge
	Efficiency of treatment, support in current goals, health insurance

and clients are factors that can make efficient and effective therapy possible or stand in the way of successful therapy outcomes. Several elements are indicated in Table 4.3 for each factor, which provides options for speech therapists to implement and integrate, and for clients to benefit from the therapeutic experience.

Another possible reason why therapy may be ineffective might be the inability of PWC to identify the sensory or musical aspects of their symptoms; they do not perceive that their speech is too fast or dysrhythmic. In these cases, audio-visual feedback (AVF) training is indicated (See Section 7.4). Finally, therapy may have started at an inappropriate or difficult time in the client's life for them to engage in a challenging therapy regimen. If this is the case, the therapist should explore other options or postpone the next appointment until a more appropriate time can be agreed upon. The speech therapist may also ask the client in these circumstances to record their speech samples monthly for identification purposes until the client is ready for change.

4.5   Analysis of recordings and questionnaires

The speech therapist will analyze the recordings and questionnaires and then decide on rate (rate adjustment), fluency, articulation, language, and the cognitive and emotional components of the disorder (see Table 4.4). Comparing the perspective of the client with the perspective of the speech therapist can

Table 4.4 Cluttering Assessment (Van Zaalen et al., 2008)

Cluttering research	Findings and interpretation
Rate	Mean articulatory rate (MAR) in SPS (in ten to 20 consecutive syllables)
	Rating of the degree of irregularity in speech output (i.e., when the pauses occur at the phrase or clause syntactical juncture)
Fluency	Percentage of typical disfluencies
	Percentage of stuttering-like disfluencies
	Stuttering Severity Instrument-4 (Riley, 2009)
Articulation	Accuracy of syllabus and word structure
	Appropriate stress patterns and prosody, the naturalness of speech, speech intelligibility
Language	Word, sentence, and story structure, cohesion and coherence of stories, pragmatics
Cognitive and emotional aspects	Feelings and attitudes toward communication
	Self-awareness of cluttering and other speech and language behaviors
Perspective	Comparison of results of speech tasks and perspectives of the speech therapist and the client on different aspects of the client's communicative behavior
	Use the CAB. Speech therapists present an overview of their findings and perspectives to the client

inform the speech therapist about the extent to which the client is aware of the disorder and their motivation to overcome it.

Speech therapist uses the assessment forms to keep track of their findings and the relationships between these findings.

4.5.1   Mean articulatory rate (MAR)

After recording the client, the speech therapist will complete the spontaneous speech analysis, reading aloud, and retelling form. These forms can be used to analyze the articulatory rate, fluency, word and sentence structures, and the use and duration of pauses. Many researchers (Hall et al., 1999; Pindzola et al., 1989) agree that articulatory rate measurements are intended to illustrate how quickly sounds are produced in consecutive speech segments, without pauses. In the assessment, the articulatory rate is primarily calculated in syllables or phonemes per second in perceptually fluent segments. Perceptually fluent productions contain no disfluencies, hesitations, or pauses longer than 250 milliseconds (Yaruss et al., 1994). Measuring the duration and counting the number of syllables is more manageable with the speech analysis software PRAAT (Boersma & Weenink, 2022). Using Praat, the client's speech can be downloaded for free over the internet and is safe to use on all systems. The assessment takes two minutes for the recording and four minutes for the analysis. When counting syllables, the speech therapist must choose between the linguistically correct word form planned before the person speaks and the actual speech motor output.

> An important question is: 'Should the speech therapist count what the client intended to say or what the client actually said?'

Based on the assumption that the client has planned a correct word form before speaking, the linguistic word form determines the articulatory rate. If the client says /library/, the number of syllables needed to produce "library" is calculated when counting the syllables. This approach is used because it is important to know how much time a person has planned for producing the word to determine whether a client has a problem in speech planning (Verhoeven et al., 2004).

Table 4.5 shows the average articulatory rate for fluent speakers of different ages. When interpreting articulatory rate scores of PWC, these rates can be used as comparison material.

Table 4.5 Standards for MAR, randomly measured in a three-minute speech sample, within sequences of ten to 20 consecutive fluent syllables (Van Zaalen et al., 2009b; Van Zaalen, 2009)

Age	Syllables per second (SPS)
6–11 years	2.5–5.0
12–22 years	2.5–5.5
23–64 years	2.5–5.3
> 65 years	2.5–4.8

A speech therapist measures the articulatory rate of an 8-year-old boy. The average of the five randomly collected measurements is 7.2 SPS. As seen in Table 4.5, this means that the average speech rate of the boy is higher than the average speech rate of his peers. But as mentioned earlier, more than the fast rate is needed to diagnose the boy with cluttering. If this boy does not simultaneously exhibit one of the three core characteristics – an excessive number of typical disfluencies or errors in pausing or impaired intelligibility –then he cannot be diagnosed with cluttering. If all three core characteristics are absent, this boy presents with tachylalia.

It should be emphasized that the MAR is only used as an indicator of rate and is necessary for the interpretation of the effect of language complexity on rate. In cluttering, there is an imbalance between rate and language formulation, which is evident in some people. However, even if their articulatory rate is still within normal limits, it may still be too fast for their speech production and monitoring system to process. This statement is especially true for people with an intellectual disability or other underlying condition. When average scores of the articulatory rate are below the norm, and there is no indication of cluttering, the condition is referred to as bradylalia. When average scores of the articulatory rate are above the norm, the condition is referred to as tachylalia, provided there are no cluttering characteristics. The procedure to determine the average articulatory rate is discussed in detail in the CAB (Van Zaalen & Reichel, 2014; Van Zaalen & Winkelman, 2009)

4.5.2   Analysis of disfluencies

Disfluencies in speaking can be analyzed by determining the number (frequency), type, and ratio between the different disfluencies. Typical disfluencies occur in the speech of all people, with or without a speech disorder.

Frequency of disfluencies

A speech sample of at least 100 and preferably 300 words is required to determine the frequency of disfluencies. It is advisable to count the typical disfluencies in a similar way to how the speech therapist counts stuttering-like disfluencies. The number of typical disfluencies indicates the extent to which the speech rate is adjusted to language planning skills. Based on studies by Eggers (2010) and Blokker et al. (2010), an average percentage of 8.97 (SD 5.5) typical disfluencies in a sample of 100 words are seen within spontaneous speech. This is not significantly different from the number of typical disfluencies when retelling a story (M = 9.17; SD 5.38), but both differ from reading a text aloud (M = 3.32; SD 2.33).

Janssen (1985), Howell and Au-Yeung (2002), and St. Louis et al. (2007) advise speech therapists to take typical disfluencies into account when evaluating fluency disorders. For example, cluttering and stuttering often coexist. Speech therapists would do well to use the modified stuttering frequency form provided in the Stuttering Severity Instrument-4 (SSI-4) (Riley, 2009), which is included as part of the Cluttering Assessment Battery. A limitation of the SSI-4 is that typical disfluencies are entirely ignored.

Types of disfluencies

Typical disfluencies (TDF) are those disfluencies that occur in spontaneous speech and occur without additional uncontrolled muscle tension; for example, word, syllable or sentence repetitions, revisions, and interjections. People are usually unaware of TDF but are aware of stuttering-like disfluencies (SLDF). SLDF are those disfluencies that interrupt the speech flow, such as tense pauses, words, syllables, or sound repetitions, prolongations

Ratio of disfluencies (RDF)

Scientific research has shown that the ratio of disfluencies (RDF) distinguishes cluttering from stuttering more than the percentages of SLDF from percentages of TDF (Van Zaalen et al., 2009b, 2009c, 2009d). The RDF is determined by dividing the percentage of TDF by the percentage of SLDF. For the interpretation of the RDF see Table 4.6. A therapist should not use the table to make a diagnosis, but it can be referred to for guiding the therapist's considerations during the differential diagnosis of cluttering.

Table 4.6 Average scores on the Stuttering Severity Instrument-4 (SSI-4) (Riley, 2009) and ratio disfluencies in a group of people with cluttering, cluttering-stuttering, and stuttering (Van Zaalen et al., 2009b)

	Cluttering	Cluttering-stuttering	Stuttering
Stuttering Severity Instrument-4	No stuttering – mild stuttering	Mild – moderate stuttering	Mild – severe stuttering
Ratio Disfluencies	RD ≥ 2.7	0 < RD > 2.7	≤ 0

4.6   Analysis of different speech conditions

The following sections describe procedures for analyzing rate, fluency, and intelligibility in different speaking conditions. Comprehensibility and intelligibility of the message are of great importance to both the speaker and the listener, but understanding is subject to perception, knowledge of the speaker and the subject, the space, and the prior knowledge of the listener. Comprehensibility and intelligibility can, therefore, hardly be measured objectively.

4.6.1   *Case history*

Immediately after obtaining a duly signed consent form, the speech therapist who is about to treat a client with cluttering must prepare a more detailed background history of the client, including the client's complaints, while recording the initial discussions with the PWC. Recordings make it possible to have an open conversation with the client before processing the initial information. For the content of the case history questions, refer to Chapter 3, Section 3.2.

4.6.2   *Spontaneous speech*

The speech therapist engages the client with cluttering in a relaxed exchange on a subject of great importance to the client. This could be explaining a video game, discussing the client's favorite sport or leisure activity, or telling a story about a recent exciting event the PWC experienced. The speech therapist must record at least ten minutes of this language sample. The language sample should be a story, not a list of events. The percentage of speaking time taken up by the speech therapist is preferably very low (less than ten percent). After all, only after about 30 to 40 seconds does the typical client switch to their automatic language, which is the language the speech therapist wants to analyze.

Experience shows that this initial conversation between the client and the speech therapist can be more spontaneous and interactive when it is informal. When the client is unaware of the recording, the speech therapist has the best chance of recording "uncontrolled" or cluttering-like speech. Such speech can also be observed when recording the interaction between a parent and a child or between an adult and a partner when the speech therapist is not in the room (Van Zaalen et al., 2008). During the speech therapist's first telephone contact with the client, the speech performance of the client can be examined by the speech therapist, who should ask questions about the symptoms of the client. The speech therapist may consider that the increased concentration of the PWC in this first contact can positively influence speech production unintentionally. If possible, the client or their parent/partner will be asked to make home recordings before the first face-to-face session with the speech therapist. This will allow the speech therapist to draw preliminary conclusions immediately at the first consultation and share them with the client.

After making the recording, the speech therapist will ask the client for their impressions of their speech performance based on this recording. The speech therapist does not immediately tell what their findings are, because a comparison of the perception of the client and the perception of the speech therapist will provide insight into the level of speech awareness of the client. It is well known that the client's speech in the first session is much more focused than is generally the case, being slightly less disfluent or unintelligible than usual (See Chapter 2, Section 2.2.10).

It can be assumed that the client also "practiced" their speech before the first visit. One way to reduce this learning effect is to ask the client in the first session to describe something they did not expect to talk about. It is advisable for speech therapists to ask something at a high level of language complexity (see Chapter 7, Section 7.2). The processing of the spontaneous speech sample, which should always be done in the presence of the client, takes about 15 minutes.

4.6.3   *Reading aloud*

The nature of the oral reading task will limit the possibilities for language formulation problems in PWC. It is advisable for speech therapists to use a reading text that includes communication between people. However, there are likely to be several errors in prosody or during word production. For example, the omission or replacement of syllables and words (especially pronouns and articles) may be evident. In addition, therapists should watch for errors in syllables and word structure, such as telescoping or guessing at words. Three measurements of at least two minutes of continuous reading of the same text should be performed (Van Zaalen, 2010). Rate, fluency, and intelligibility are measured using the Cluttering Assessment Battery. Reading aloud and spontaneous speech are evaluated similarly, making it easy to compare the effect of the task on rate, fluency, and intelligibility.

Because the level of the reading material can affect the severity of cluttering, speech therapists must present appropriate reading material that varies in complexity to their clients. For example, the more difficult passages containing more multisyllabic words and more linguistically complex sentences can trigger more cluttering-like behaviors than the less difficult passages. But the moment the client becomes aware of the difficulty and increases their focus, the cluttering characteristics will decrease.

We also recommend asking the client to read one prepared passage and one without preparation, to enable the therapist to compare the results of both measurements. Compared to people who don't clutter, PWC who read the same material four times in a row exhibit less focused attention during repeated measurements. The result of less attention is audible and manifested by an increase in guess reading, telescopic reading of multisyllabic words, and disfluencies compared to previous measurements, especially when a reading text is significantly below the reading level of the PWC. If that happens, it is an indication of possible cluttering. Because the level of auditory monitoring in the PWC while speaking is less than normal, the speech therapist should ask the PWC to evaluate their intelligibility, rate, and fluency immediately after reading the correct text.

The distinction between cluttered reading and dyslexia

It is well-known that reading aloud with headphones on (increased auditory feedback) compensates for weak monitoring during speech and, thereby, reduces moments of incomprehensibility, disfluencies, and reading errors. This is where the cluttering reader stands out from a reader with dyslexia.

Reading provides important information about the emotional component of the speech disorder. For example, a therapist should consider whether PWC feel comfortable reading. Are the PWC under the impression that they can better control their speech while reading than during spontaneous speech? Comparing the client's perceptions with the perceptions of the speech therapist provides diagnostic data and the first insight into the client's symptom awareness. This can be confrontational, but it is also a therapeutically valuable experience for the client.

4.6.4   Retelling a story

The Wallet Story is specifically designed to collect information about voice output when less attention is paid to story developing compared to spontaneous speech. Such a goal is achieved because the speech therapist provides both the story structure and the sentence structure to the client. If auditory memory is normal, such an approach will help the client to remember the story structure and parts of the sentence structure. This concept is developed by Van Zaalen and Bochane (2007) based on the principles underlying the Bus Story, and the story construction test of the Arizona Battery for Communication Disorders of Dementia (ABCD). The Bus Story can be used for children under 12 years old. After retelling the story, the speech therapist analyzes the components of the story, the articulatory rate, the ratio of disfluencies, and the structure of the sentences. Assessing the components and speech output of a story in a structured setting makes it possible for the therapist to compare the results of the client's analysis with those of other people and the client analyzing their speech output in different speaking contexts.

Many speech therapists have noted that PWC have difficulties in storytelling. PWC are often tempted to provide more detailed information than necessary. They also need help maintaining the storyline. However, these impressions are not supported by empirical research. On the contrary, in retelling the aforementioned Wallet Story, PWC diverted to side issues similar to people with learning difficulties and typical speakers, adding irrelevant information that did not belong to the story (noise). A study by Van Zaalen et al. (2009b) indicated that PWC are distinguished from PWS by their adding side issues and making additional comments that are not relevant to the story.

A comparison of the scores for rate, fluency, and intelligibility gives the speech therapist more information about the influence of language formulation on the quality of the speech of PWS. For example, sometimes PWC can imitate or use complex language structures while retelling a story, but these PWC have difficulties doing so in spontaneous speech. The errors in the language formulation in those cases are not related to a lack of language production skills, but to a lack of formulation skills during spontaneous speech with a fast articulatory rate. In such a case, working on sentence structure would be less effective for changing speech output than working on the speech rate and phrasing.

4.6.5 *Writing and handwriting*

Reading and writing are the highest levels of speech and language development (Van Zaalen & Bochane, 2007). Based on unpublished pilot research by Luchtmeijer and Van Zaalen, the articulatory rate appears strongly correlated with the writing speed. PWC, who produce many typical disfluencies in their speech tend to do so when they need to write something down quickly. On the other hand, PWC who have poor speech intelligibility tend to write in such small letters, including the night candle effect (see Chapter 2, Section 2.2.6), that the handwriting becomes difficult to read (see Figure 4.2).

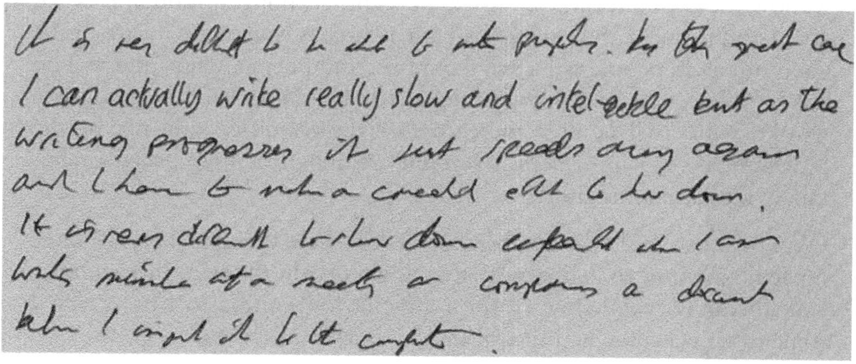

Figure 4.2 Examples of writing and writing for phonological and syntactic cluttering

---

A sample of Peter's "unguarded" typing,
telling some of his personal story:

I have had problems for many years, which started when I was at schol as far as I can remember, reading out in calss was one ot the problems, teacxhers would riducoue me for speaking funy, one wuol,d ay to me "speak ip bioy don't mumble", felow puoils woueld taunt me, no one understod me properly, I msde freinds but don't knwo how myana.

I woked hard, I was quiet, and fiound it hadr to tlak to people about some thisnhgs, adn this has hapend al my life and has held up my ecducation and employemnt. Even wehn I statred work people used to taunt me becasue I taklekd funny! I wa sbulied at scgol and at work, no one seemded to care. Life was so frustrating and intimidating, I had no idea that I had a porblem tlike \I know today, if I as awatre of tnis and the teacjhers ot my partent had adddressed this, i could myabwe had some help, hmmm, maybe not, no one knwe about clutering in those days, but it oculd have ben found that I had a comunication pronb;lem.

I have treid al my life to please peole, I was told thaty I would never do any god in life and I tried to probve evrybody worng, I ewnt into busines in the 1970's and I struggeld to hold run a business sucsesfuly, I was not harfd enought to condunt a bisusiness proplery, nad fater mnay eyars I had to amdnit defeat, I packed it al up and went back to working fro zomseone else. At least I got pasid on a Friday every week.

Whne working in the garages I was a motoer vehicle techniician and was god at my job, it would have been goukd ofr promotion, but each time I apliead for poromotion I was told dthat my spech was not suiyatbale for speaing to custommomers and for teh many aplications I made in fiddefernt companies thaye gave me the sdame story.

After tears of feeling insecure, differnt, isolated and excluded, I know Kknow the comndition I have, which is clutteroimng, although it is not cured and nebver can be as fra as I am aware, at lwast I am aware of the conditini aadn people wil learn from tihs, and poepke who sufer as I do wil be able t undrestand what they ahve, the amin thinsg is, peiopokle worlkd wide awil be able to reecognise the condition and maybe the ptofessionals can impement a suitable treainhg/teacjhing athen evebntaualy a treatment regime.

Ok, nuffs. enough! eh? the above sentences were typed as I type, I have made no attempt to delibertaly slow down or edit the text, this sentence is deliberately typed slow (waht a difficult job!) and aslo I have edited some of it, as even when typing slowly, I make mistakes.

Figure 4.3 Typed English text by a person with syntactic cluttering.

Similarly, to linguistic weaknesses, poor handwriting is one of the earliest behaviors associated with cluttering. Some older PWC use the compensatory strategy of printing out their written texts. It is recommended to ask PWC to write, both in script and by print, for comparison purposes. Spelling errors can reflect problems in the speech domain, so the client should be asked to write a short paragraph, after which the speech therapist should look for sloppy or illegible writing, poor spelling, improperly constructed grammar, and transposition and omission of letters as evidence of cluttering-related behaviors.

Handwriting skills and their motor-perceptual connections in the brain can positively influence reading ability. Learning to write letters by hand generates cerebral sensorimotor representations. These motor programs are elicited by writing the learned letters. In addition, Longcamp et al. (2011) also discovered that with the help of fMRI these stored motor programs are activated when reading letters, i.e., when passively observing them. However, this was only noted if the letters had previously been written by hand. This proves that a close functional relationship exists between reading and handwriting movements (Marquardt et al., 2016). It is, therefore, conceivable that the problems that PWC experience in text comprehension can be partly remediated by improvements in handwriting and vice versa. However, this assumption needs to be examined further. Handwriting speed can be determined using the Handwriting Speed Test (Wallen et al., 1996). In this test, the client is asked to write a standardized sentence ten times in quick succession over a pre-set time period. The manuscript will then be analyzed, consulting the handwriting observation lists of Van Hartingsveldt et al. (2010).

According to Van Hartingsveldt et al., (2010), the speech therapist must analyze characteristics such as fluency in movement, the amplitude of the movement, the pressure on the paper, spatial positioning, readability, and writing speed. If the client is found to have severe graphomotor problems, for example, illegible handwriting, this should be considered when planning therapeutic intervention. Consulting a physical therapist or occupational therapist is recommended in those cases.

Cluttering can also be observed in typed text, as shown in the example of Peter in Figure 4.3.

4.6.6 *Screening Phonological Accuracy*

Each speaker can be examined for potential problems in speech-motor control and phonological encoding. Speech motor control problems in stuttering can be identified by using the OMAS (Riley & Riley, 1985; Van Zaalen & Winkelman, 2009) (See Chapter 3, Sections 3.10 and Chapter 4, Section 4.6.7). If a client is unintelligible or mispronounces multisyllabic words, it is advisable to assess phonological planning at a word or sentence level and to examine speech motor skills. To assess the phonological planning and execution skills of PWC, the SPA has been developed (Van Zaalen et al., 2011)

PWC often exhibit abnormal phonological encoding skills at the word level. Their inhibition problem prevents them from adjusting their speech rate to the higher level of planning skills in low-frequency multisyllabic words. Low-frequency words take a longer lexicon retrieval time pickup time than high-frequency words. Frequently used words can be retrieved much faster based on linguistic motor memory. Words that are infrequently used should be planned before execution starts.

Although this planning takes time, PWC are "forced" to speak fast, as they do not have enough planning time. PWC complete syllable planning at the same time as they are producing the word. On repeated attempts, unlike typical speakers, PWC cannot benefit from the motor plan of a previously well-executed production. Although fluent speakers are able to produce the SPA words three times fast, equally, and intelligibly, PWC plan for each of the three sequences by making three separate attempts. Meanwhile, the SPA is available in Dutch, English, German, French, Norwegian, Polish, and Finnish.

4.6.7   Oral Motor Assessment Scale

The OMAS at the sound level was initially developed by Riley and Riley (1985) and was later modified to digital recording and analysis by Van Zaalen (2009). The OMAS is the most effective tool to rule out oral-motor problems and to explain intelligibility problems. The OMAS not only assesses the rate, but it also precisely shows the extent of the problem that can provide insight into the client's oral-motor skills. The client's ability to adjust their syllable sequencing (temporal order) and syntactic formulation skills (grammatical order) to the speech rate is an indication of what needs to be improved. Information about the articulatory rate at which PWC can produce sound sequences without linguistic content can help to determine the ideal articulatory rate for that person. The articulatory rate that PWC can maintain to control their syntactic planning and motor movements can be identified as a goal for facilitating an appropriate speech rate in therapy. A MAR depends on different speaking situations or on the level of language complexity. Therefore, the mean rate at which language is produced in the OMAS task should be considered the absolute maximum mean rate level. If a person can only speak clearly in contexts with low language demands, the speech rate should be even slower in situations with higher language complexity.

Table 4.7 shows various aspects of speech-motor control (Riley & Riley, 1985).

Table 4.7 Speech motor control

Aspect	Variable	Correct production	Incorrect production
Accuracy	Distortion	A good articulation position & appropriate strength	In voiced sounds, the voice onset is not well adjusted to the articulatory movements: voice onset time (VOT)
	Voicing	Normal voicing	Voiced sounds are produced as voiceless, and vice versa
Smooth flow	Coarticulation	A gradual transition from one sound to another	Additional pauses between syllables or tense vocal onset
	Flow	Equal rhythm and normal stress	Dysrhythmic production
	Telescoping	Correct number of syllables	Deletion of syllables within a sequence (for example: 'pa-ta-ka' produced as /paka-paka/)
	Sequencing	A correct sequence of sounds or syllables	The order of the syllables is different (for example, 'pataka' becomes /pakata/; 'pata' becomes /pa-at/)
Rate	Syllables per second	Mean rate measured over three attempts of ten syllables	Extremely slow production (below 3 SPS), possibly with additional pauses

The characteristics of speech-motor control are related to verbal-motor elements, such as syllables, and not to nonverbal elements like tongue movements, lip rounding, and jaw movements.

When Edwin (22.3 years) talks about his vacation; a mean rate of 6.0 SPS is sufficient for the motor control of his speech output. When Edwin wants to comment on the additional policy of the swimming pool, the rate of 6.0 SPS leads to a high frequency of telescoping and typical disfluencies. Edwin produced "pataka" at a rate of 6.5 SPS. After a suggestion from the speech therapist, Edwin lowered his speech rate (measured at 5.1 SPS), showing that he can control his speech rate once again.

4.6.8 *Brief Cluttering and Stuttering Questionnaire (BCSQ)*

The ten-item qualitative BCSQ, created by Reichel (2010), is the first interview protocol for therapists and clients with combined cases of cluttering and stuttering to understand the impact of both disorders on clients' lives. It examines the responses of such clients regarding various aspects of both disorders, such as the effects of nègative stigma, the influence of both disorders on each other, a comparison of the affective aspect of both disorders, which language (primary or secondary) is affected more by cluttering, and which by stuttering. In addition, BCSQ attempts to ascertain whether clients may have syntactic or phonological subtypes of cluttering based on clients' responses to the question: "What interferes more with your communication? Planning and formulating thoughts or fast and unclear speech?" Difficulties in planning and formulating thoughts indicate syntactic cluttering, while fast and unclear speech indicates phonological cluttering. This questionnaire can also be used as a clinical tool for developing client-centered interventions with consideration of their priorities in the treatment of both disorders (Exum et al., 2010).

4.6.9   *Speech analysis with the PRAAT software*

Objective acoustic speech analysis is not often performed within the speech pathology community. Assessment of speech generally occurs based on perceptual findings. It is possible that the speech of a client is perceived as too fast by one speech therapist, and it can be perceived as normal by another speech therapist. This client does not benefit from this difference in perceptions of the two therapists, as this difference can get in the way of a correct diagnosis. Clinical decisions are best when made based on objective measurements; for example, when using speech analysis software such as PRAAT (Boersma & Weenink, 2022). Chapters 6 and 7 explain the use of Talk in exercises; Score forms and test instruments are described in this chapter.

As mentioned earlier in Chapter 3, PRAAT is a speech analysis and synthesis software written by Paul Boersma and David Weenink from the Department of Phonetics at the University of Amsterdam. The software can be downloaded for free from www.fon.hum.uva.nl/praat. A user manual can also be found on the same website. The program is constantly being improved and updated. PRAAT assists with speech analysis spectral pitch, formant and intensity analysis, jitter, and shimmer), speech synthesis (pitch, formant and intensity, and articulatory synthesis), listening experiments (identification and discrimination tests), and speech manipulation (change of pitch and duration contours). The digital speech analysis helps make the measurements objective, and it provides insight into the speech of PWC. In addition, the speech analysis procedure can serve as a therapeutic feedback tool. The installation of the software takes only two minutes. Most PWC who are eight years of age or older can use PRAAT after one or two ten-minute instructional sessions. PRAAT is beneficial for analyses, for diagnostics, and for the treatment/monitoring of speech for PWC. This software is used worldwide in speech therapy scientific research.

PRAAT is an excellent tool for online therapy, especially if the PWC and the speech therapist both work on their own versions of PRAAT or share a screen with each other. PRAAT works with audio files, preferably saved as a *.wav file or a *.mp4 file. Files recorded with a phone can be shared via platforms like WhatsApp. To analyze the files recorded with a phone, they need to be converted to a *.wav file. Sharing sound files recorded with a computer is best done through websites like WeTransfer.

4.6.10   *Cluttering self-assessment checklists*

Self-evaluation of speech is possible using various tools or instructions. Self-evaluation provides insight into the cognitive and emotional factors of cluttering in PWC. Instruments explicitly developed for other speech therapy disorders have been adapted and, in some cases, standardized for use with cluttering. An example of this is the Speech Situation Checklist, created by Brutten and Janssen (1981) and adapted to cluttering. The impact of cluttering on a person's life can be assessed using the Wright & Ayre Stuttering Self-Rating Profile (WASSP) (Wright & Ayre, 2000) as modified for cluttering. Some of the WASSP's questions relate to the physical aspects of disfluencies. When these questions are related to cluttering behavior, comparisons can be made between the observations of the speech therapist and those of the client. The modification of the Overall Assessment of the Speaker's Experience of Stuttering (OASES) (Yaruss & Quesal, 2010) for cluttering is under development. The OASES, as developed for stuttering, is not helpful for cluttering. The speech therapist may ask the client to assess her own speech during various recorded tasks, which should then be compared with the speech therapist's feedback. A five-point rating scale helps (ranging from one: normal, without complaints; to five: severely disfluent or severely unintelligible) to judge the recorded samples on each of the major areas of the client's speech and language.

4.7   Differential diagnosis

Differential diagnosis refers to the diagnosis in which a choice is made between closely related alternatives. The next chapter discusses differential diagnostics between cluttering and other disorders or conditions, such as stuttering, learning difficulties, tachylalia, developmental apraxia of speech, specific language disorders, neurogenic cluttering, and dysarthria. Furthermore, Chapter 5 discusses the prevalence of cluttering in several disorders and syndromes where the individual also speaks too fast, too slow, or inconsistently, such as people with Down syndrome, ASD, fragile X syndrome, Tourette's syndrome, NF1, and ADHD.

Pure cluttering occurs in some PWC. They experience cluttering without other disorders. People with pure cluttering can also use their fast movements and processes and lack of inhibition for other activities in life, such as studying (studying multiple subjects at the same time), sports (endurance), or development of intelligence (above-average intelligence level). It is striking that among PWC, there is a significant percentage of people with a high IQ and a successful social career. They have been able to turn their fast and uninhibited behavior into their strength. In the literature, little or no attention has been paid to the positive aspects of the cluttering. This still needs additional research, which will focus on the person's potential rather than limitations.

Cluttering, as referenced above, often coexists with other disorders or with various syndromes, such as stuttering, articulation disorders, and learning disabilities. The available literature suggests that an essential difference between cluttering and other forms of speech disorders is based on the level of preparedness of the speaker for expressing intended messages. Typical speakers know what they want to say and use appropriate linguistic and motor planning and execution. PWS know what they intend to say but have motor difficulty producing different words. PWC do not necessarily know in advance everything they want to say (or how to say it), but they start or continue talking anyway. PWS, however, present with blockages, prolongations, and sound and syllable repetitions. Frequent characteristics of cluttering and of individuals with syndromes or disorders, such as NF1 or learning difficulties, are excessive but typical disfluencies.

PWC often exceed the normal qualitative and quantitative limits of changes in phonemes and tend to remove or neutralize syllables that standard speakers do not neutralize, especially in fast speech. Although symptoms of ADD are often considered indicative of cluttering, individuals diagnosed with ADHD/ADD do not necessarily have cluttering. Specific learning disabilities (SLD) have been reported to be associated with cluttering, particularly problems with oral expression, reading, writing, handwriting, and music; however, confirmatory data for these observations are anecdotal and not yet sufficiently substantiated in a scientific manner.

4.7.1   Differential diagnostic criteria

Eisenson (1986) described cluttering as a "cousin" of stuttering, in which both conditions stem from the same family tree. Historically, cluttering was considered the same disorder as stuttering (Georgieva, 2010; Van Riper, 1970). Several experts from Germany (deHirsch, 1970; Freund, 1966; Froeschels, 1946) and Austria (Weiss, 1964) believed that cluttering causes stuttering. DeHirsch (1970) pointed out that children with profligate behavior whose language systems are immature and disorganized are likely to become stutterers due to emotional conflict and stress.

Speech therapists should conduct diagnostic assessments within their clinics to evaluate the speech output of PWC. To plan effective treatment, it is important to distinguish between types and subtypes of disorders, while at the same time excluding potentially coexisting disorders. A differential diagnosis in fluency disorders is also important for identifying cluttering-like or stuttering components and, at the same time, understanding the effect of rate on the speech output of PWC. As described above, there are many syndromes in

Assessment instruments 97

which disfluencies or problems with intelligibility occur. A thorough assessment is needed under different speaking conditions to distinguish between the various disorders and syndromes.

> Making a diagnosis based only on one or two symptoms is insufficient for all communication disorders. It is the profile of speaking behavior in different circumstances that provides speech therapists with answers about the underlying problems of their clients with cluttering. Only a complete profile will lead to the correct diagnosis.

Note: symptoms may change during speech and language intervention. A component may be overlooked in a person with severe blockages since it may prevent the person from speaking without inhibitions. It is also possible that PWC may suffer from severe negative reactions to speaking based on their communication experiences, but do not express these thoughts at the beginning of therapy because they are unaware of the relationship between their speech problems and these negative thoughts. As previously noted, Chapter 5 delves deeper into the similarities and differences between cluttering and other communication disorders.

4.7.2 Diagnostic markers

As described in Chapter 1, cluttering is characterized by an articulatory rate that is too fast or too variable, resulting in a high frequency of typical disfluencies and errors in pausing or word structure. However, not every fast speaker is considered a person with cluttering; some non-cluttering people also make mistakes in pausing or word structure or have a high frequency of "normal" disfluencies. In other words, no single characteristic independently justifies a diagnosis of cluttering, unlike the different responses to changes in language complexity that characterize cluttering. Van Heeswijk (2011) has shown that the PWC produce significantly more typical disfluencies and word structure errors than fluent individuals; but this also applies to people with intellectual disabilities, dysarthria, Parkinson's disease, or some types of aphasia. The extent to which the underlying mechanism for the disfluencies in the above-mentioned syndromes is similar to the underlying mechanism for cluttering (if at all) is not intrinsically a diagnostic marker for cluttering.

When the PWC do not adjust their speech rate to the linguistic complexity of multisyllabic words, then word structure errors can easily occur. The most obvious errors are sequencing errors and overcoarticulation (telescoping). When producing complex multisyllabic segments three times in a row, planning normally takes place before production. When the pre-production planning takes place, each production is carried out separately according to the same plan. When planning is completed during production, each production is different. The SPA referenced previously (Van Zaalen et al., 2011; see Section 4.6.6) is sensitive to these processes and can be used as a diagnostic tool for identifying phonological cluttering.

4.8 Summary

This chapter has discussed the different components of the Cluttering Assessment Battery: first, the variables to be assessed, and then the content of the diagnostic assessment. The diagnostic assessment is one of the components to recognize the change readiness of the PWC. Subsequently, the analyses within the various speaking tasks are reviewed, which are associated with differential diagnosis.

5 Cluttering and other disorders

5.1 Cluttering and other disorders with an irregular speech rate

Cluttering is a phenomenon that has been associated with a range of disorders and syndromes. It is important to note that a relatively limited amount of research has been conducted that investigates the occurrence of cluttering in individuals with or without other disorders. As such, the data discussed in the following sections need further validation through rigorous scientific research. This section will discuss the disorders that are also known for their irregular rate: dyslexia (section 5.1.1); language developmental disorder or language processing disorder (5.1.2); stuttering (5.1.3); ASD (5.1.4); ADHD/ ADD (5.1.5); and neurogenic disorders (5.1.6). Section 5.2 will discuss the disorders known for their excessively fast or slow speech rate.

5.1.1 Cluttering and dyslexia

The latest definition of the Dyslexia Fund Foundation International Dyslexia Association (NY) is:

> "Dyslexia is a specific learning disability that is characterized by a persistent problem in learning accurate and smooth reading and/or spelling at the word level, which is not the result of environmental factors and/or a physical, neurological, or general intellectual disability."

> "Dyslexia is a specific learning disability that is neurobiological in origin. It is characterized by difficulties with accurate and/or fluent word recognition and by poor spelling and decoding abilities. These difficulties typically result from a deficit in the phonological component of language that is often unexpected in relation to other cognitive abilities and the provision of effective classroom instruction. Secondary consequences may include problems in reading comprehension and reduced reading experience that can impede growth of vocabulary and background knowledge."

DOI: 10.4324/9781003460558-7

Based on new knowledge by Taylor and Vestergaard (2022), dyslexia is considered not as a disorder but as a form of neurodiversity characterized by a unique way of processing, storing, and reproducing information with characteristic weaknesses and strengths. Dyslexia and cluttering are both characterized by persistent problems with reading aloud. A significant difference between cluttering and dyslexia is that the problems in reading associated with cluttering temporarily disappear with increased auditory feedback; for example, this occurs when an individual speaks into a microphone and hears the speech back through headphones. This is never the case with dyslexia. While the differences between reading aloud with and without headphones/microphones are apparent to listeners, PWC do not consciously notice the difference while reading. When listening to a recording, the differences are noticed by PWC. In the case of people with dyslexia, errors also appear during writing and reading, whereas in the case of people with cluttering, errors often disappear.

5.1.2   *Cluttering and Specific Language Impairment*

A specific language impairment (SLI) is a neurobiological developmental disorder. This means that language is less well processed in the brain. For example, a child with SLI has significant difficulty talking or understanding language. As a result, language and speech development is different for them than it is for their peers.

Children with SLI:

- hear well;
- learn their mother tongue slowly and laboriously;
- have normal intelligence;
- have difficulty remembering sounds and words;
- have difficulty with grammar;
- have difficulty dealing with emotions;
- need help planning sentences.

Cluttering disrupts the fluency of the language, affecting all communication modalities (e.g., reading, writing, rhythm, and musicality) and behavior in general. Myers and St. Louis (2007) and van Zaalen et al. (2009) conclude that PWC demonstrate normal scores on language tests. The more complex the message of PWC, the more likely it is that problems with language formulation will occur. Based on clinical observation, the language problems of PWC do not necessarily indicate a language disorder. The language problems of PWC disappear when they speak slowly or when they write.

People with language production problems, such as semantic permutations, difficulties finding words, or syntax problems, can be differentiated from PWC. The main distinction is that production problems of people with

SLI do not disappear when they speak more slowly or write. Instead, they must develop the necessary grammatical construction skills or lexical selection (word-finding) strategies.

5.1.3 Cluttering and stuttering

Cluttering is a disorder that is similar to stuttering but is also different in many ways. Cluttering and stuttering, when occurring at the same time, are called *balbuties e paraphrasia praecipe* in Latin (Freund, in Weiss, 1964). These two disorders were first described as comorbid in the early part of the last century by Scripture (1912), although the first detailed description of these two coexisting disorders was made over a century ago when many speech therapists knew little about cluttering. They confused cluttering with stuttering or other disorders (Ward, 2018). St. Louis et al. (1985) explored the differences between stuttering and cluttering symptoms. They found that people with combined cluttering and stuttering produce a high frequency of disfluencies. PWC produce significantly fewer repetitions of sounds and syllables, prolongations, and tense pauses than PWS. In PWC, the speech distortions appear to be caused by an attempt to gain time for linguistic planning. The speech of PWS is characterized by tension and a struggle to produce what was already planned.

Cluttering and cluttering-stuttering differ from stuttering by the following characteristics:

1. A fast or variable articulatory rate.
2. Weak speech motor control in multisyllabic words.
3. A high ratio of normal disfluencies.
4. Abnormal rate adjustment to linguistic complexity.
5. Focused attention makes speech better.
6. Relaxation increases speech disruptions.

All six characteristics that distinguish cluttering from stuttering are discussed below.

1 A fast or variable articulatory rate

Experience shows that PWC are not able to control their speech rate for longer than 40 seconds. This is especially true in speech conditions with high language complexity or when the person is significantly tired.

2 Weak speech motor control in multisyllabic words

PWC, especially those with phonological cluttering, have great difficulty maintaining appropriate syllable structure when producing complex multisyllabic words at a fast rate. This is especially true for low-frequency words (see Chapter 4, Section 4.6.6). PWS also need assistance in performing this task. They may have trouble initiating speech, but their word structure remains intact.

3   *A high ratio of typical disfluencies*

The ratio of disfluencies is defined as the relationship between the frequency of typical disfluencies to stuttering-like disfluencies (See Chapter 3, Section 3.6). PWC typically produce seven times more typical disfluencies than stuttering-like disfluencies. In cases of PWS, the ratio of disfluencies is always below three and often even below 1 (see Table 4.6 in Chapter 4).

4   *No rate adjustment to linguistic complexity*

It turns out that people with syntactic cluttering cannot adequately adjust their speech rate to the linguistic demands of the moment. When comparing the mean articulatory rate (MAR) in various speaking situations, the mean rate varies by less than 1.0 SPS. PWS, on the other hand, can adjust their articulatory rate in different linguistic contexts. The difference in the articulatory rate between speaking situations in those who can adjust their rate usually ranges between 1.0 and 3.3 SPS (Van Zaalen & Winkelman, 2009).

5   *Focused attention makes speech better.*

While PWC present better speech output when focused on their speech, additional attention to speech in PWS usually creates increased tension, making speech output more labored and disfluent.

6   *Relaxation increases speech disruptions*

In cases of PWS, relaxation has a positive effect on speech output, reducing instances of stuttering-like disfluencies. On the other hand, in cases of PWC, relaxation exacerbates their challenges, leading to more instances of fast, unintelligible, or disorganized speech. Therefore, when communicating with close relatives and friends, a relaxed environment leads to fewer instances of speech disruptions for PWS, while relaxation results in more speech disruptions for PWC.

Cluttering and stuttering have multiple similarities.

1. fear of speech
2. fear of specific words
3. underachievement in society
4. problems in social encounters
5. coping with a negative stigma

Below we will discuss these five differentiating characteristics in more detail.

1   *Fear of speech*

Fear of speech or communication apprehension arises when people feel that their message will not come across to the listener correctly or are concerned as to whether the message being conveyed is of sufficient value to share with others. Contrary to what many speech therapists believe, communication apprehension is present in combined cases of cluttering and stuttering. Both types of disfluent speakers are afraid of the listener's reactions. In PWS this fear is related to the fear of getting stuck while speaking (fear of stuttering). PWC can develop a fear of not being understood. The extent to which this fear can develop is the same for both PWS and PWC.

2   Fear of words

Fear of words in cluttering is often related to the difficulties that PWC experience when reading aloud or in producing multisyllabic words. Fear of words in stuttering is mainly linked to specific sounds or sound combinations in which PWS are not sure whether their motor output will be easy or comfortable. PWS may experience difficulties producing words that begin with a particular sound, e.g., plosives or vowels. They may also develop a fear of words that they tended to stutter on in the past.

3   Underachievement in society

Younger PWC and PWS often need help with reading aloud because their speaking problem reduces the chances for high-level performance. Speakers with stuttering and cluttering can fail to live up to their potential in many areas of life because of their speech difficulties. For example, avoiding a search for better employment can contribute to underachievement. In addition, a job requiring many phone calls or social interactions can be difficult for someone with cluttering or stuttering.

4   Problems in social encounters

PWC and PWS can develop a fear of meeting new people because they are concerned about how they will be perceived. PWC may need assistance to express their thoughts intelligibly and coherently during a team meeting. They often deal with inappropriate answers because the listener did not understand the PWC correctly. PWS may avoid words in conversation and, thus, convey different messages than intended. For example, when ordering food, they might say, "four big macs, please," when only three are desired. Some listeners are startled by stuttering and do not know how to hide their reaction to stuttering. This may come across as a lack of interest in what the PWS is saying.

Gabriella, 34: "It is so difficult for me to pronounce the name of the deceased correctly that I have decided to give up my job as a funeral director and become an ambulance driver."

Table 5.1 Characteristics of different disorders

Linguistic and psychological factors	Cluttering	Stuttering	Learning difficulties	ADD
MAR	Fast and/or irregular	Slow to medium	Normal	Normal to fast
Ratio disfluencies (NDF-SDF) in a monologue or retelling a story	Fast, especially NDF	High, especially SDF	High, especially NDF	High, especially NDF
Pauses	Too few, too short, or in linguistically inappropriate places	Too many and too long	Many pauses	Too short, in linguistically normal places
Adjusting rate to language complexity	No	Yes	Yes	No
Errors in word structure	Possible	No	Possible	Possible
Possible causes of impaired sentence structure	Sentence formulation under time pressure causes procrastination	Avoidance behavior	Sentence formulation underdeveloped	Absent
Focus makes speaking:	Better	Worse	Better	Better
Relaxation makes speaking:	Worse	Better	Better	Better
Speaking a foreign language:	Better	Vary	Worse	Better
Reading aloud a well-known text is:	Worse	Usually better, but worse in case of fear of speaking	Better	Worse
Reading an unknown text aloud is:	Better	Worse	Mostly worse	Mostly worse
Fear of communication	Possible	Possible	Absent	Absent
Awareness of symptoms during speech	Usually not	Usually present	Usually not	Present
Awareness of communication problem	Often	Usually yes	Absent	Absent
Word fear mainly in cases of:	Multisyllabic words	Mostly emotionally loaded	Absent	Absent
Sound fear	Absent	Frequent, varying between individuals	Absent	Absent

5 Dealing with a negative stigma

It is well known that the general public negatively stigmatizes PWC and PWS. For example, a study by St. Louis et al. (2011) found that respondents from four countries believe that PWC can be nervous, irritable, anxious, or shy and cannot work satisfactorily in jobs that require a significant amount of talking. When asked which disorder, between cluttering or stuttering, is stigmatized more negatively, some respondents to the previously mentioned BCSQ answered as follows (Exum et al., 2010): "People stigmatize cluttering and stuttering in different ways." "With stuttering, it's a pity/amused look, but with cluttering, it's a confused look or the long silent pause on the other end of the phone. And both disorders draw an emotional reaction, whether it's laughter or tears, it's a reaction that you never forget." "If stuttering is mostly associated with speech, cluttering, due to its unusual nature, is often associated with non-coherent thinking, a low IQ, absence of cognitive skills, low emotional intelligence, etc." "Inability to express the thoughts effortlessly and explicitly causes puzzled listeners' facial expressions and comments."

Table 5.1 gives an overview of the characteristics of different disorders with overlapping characteristics (Van Zaalen & Winkelman, 2014).

5.1.4 Autism spectrum disorder

Autism spectrum disorder (ASD) is a developmental disorder. Many experts believe that ASD is an information-processing disorder. People with autism often have difficulties with socializing and communication. They are also more sensitive or less sensitive than most people to internal and external stimuli, which makes them more likely to become overstimulated (Autisme Spectrum Centrum, 2022). Little is known about the relationship between cluttering and ASD. There is a paucity of research regarding the speech of people with ASD, which indicates that cluttering-like speech is not a frequent symptom in people with ASD. However, a higher incidence of cluttering symptoms appears in this group compared to the control group (Scaler Scott, 2011). Speech therapists who work with children with ASD often say, "I see many children with a diagnosis of ASDs that have other comorbid disorders." An ASD diagnosis can be confused with a diagnosis of cluttering. The similarities can be misleading, especially when the lack of symptom awareness is considered merely a cluttering symptom. Children diagnosed with ASD cannot take the listener's perspective, which might be confused with the abnormal pragmatic skills of PWC during fast speech. Also, the sudden transition from one topic to another, often considered a symptom of cluttering, is a frequent behavior of children with ASD. For example, children with Pervasive Developmental Disorder – Not Otherwise Specified (PDD-NOS) suffer from chaotic thinking and lack insight when processing information.

Studies examining individuals with autistic characteristics (Shields, 2010; Thacker & Austen, 1996) and those with Asperger's syndrome (Scaler Scott, 2008; Scaler Scott et al., 2007) suggest that cluttering is a condition that speech therapists should consider a potential co-existing disorder when evaluating the communication pattern of individuals with ASD (Scott & Cummings, 2017).

5.1.5 *Attention deficit hyperactivity disorder (ADHD)*

Although symptoms of ADHD (attention-deficit disorder, predominantly hyperactive-impulsive type) and ADD (attention-deficit/hyperactivity disorder, predominantly inattentive type) are often considered indicative of cluttering, individuals diagnosed with ADHD/DD do not necessarily suffer from cluttering (Ward, 2018, van Borsel et al., 2008). People with ADHD/ADD have an average to high MAR. Their ratio of disfluencies is high in favor of typical disfluencies, while appropriately placed pauses are often too short. Similarly to the experiences of PWC, people with ADHD/ADD find that increased attention to communication improves their speech, while relaxation worsens their speech. Fifteen participants with cluttering, as described in a study by St. Louis and Schulte (2011), exhibited irregularities in the attention subsection of the ADD questionnaire. Alm (2011) notes that PWC exhibit opposite responses to dopaminergic medications compared to individuals with ADHD/ADD, possibly indicating the presence of another type of attention deficit dysregulation found in the same attention system. No general differences in communication characteristics between ADHD/ADD and cluttering have been demonstrated in scientific literature to date. Some patients diagnosed with ADHD/ADD described experiencing "multiple tracks" of thought. These thought tracks are experienced simultaneously and sometimes in quick succession, switching between two or more different subjects. An external observer can describe these thought patterns as internal distractibility or as difficulty in focusing on a topic in conversation (Jerome, 2003). This phenomenon of having multiple tracks of thought is not typical for cluttering.

A study by Jang and Shin (2021) examining the disfluency of children with ADHD, stuttering, and controls showed that the children diagnosed with ADHD produced significantly more typical disfluencies in spontaneous speech than controls. These differences were not found in the reading tasks. The typical disfluencies found were mainly interjections, word or phrase repetitions, and revisions (see Table 5.2). This study also indicated that the speech rate of the children with ADHD was lower than that of the children who stutter, but the authors did not clearly explain how they calculated the speech rate.

The disfluencies referred to above disrupted the assessment of the rate; therefore, contrary to what Jang and Shin found, the articulatory rate is commonly used today instead of the speech rate. Notably, all the above-mentioned

Table 5.2 Disfluencies in children with ADHD (Jang & Shin, 2021)

	ADHD	Stuttering	Control group		
	M (SD)	M (SD)	M (SD)	F	Post-hoc
Interjection	5.87 (4.98)	10.27 (5.66)	1.13 (1.36)	16.02	c<a<b
Phrases/words repetitions	.87 (1.41)	1.93 (1.44)	.27 (.59)	7.29	c<b
Modification/ incomplete phrase	3.60 (1.99)	3.47 (3.14)	1.07 (1.09)	6.09	c<a
Hesitation	2.00 (2.65)	1.40 (1.88)	.40 (.74)	2.65	
Part word repetitions	1.80 (1.26)	7.87 (6.78)	.60 (.91)	14.10	a,c<b
One syllable repetitions	.13 (.35)	.80 (1.37)	.06 (.26)	3.56	c<b
Disrhythmic phonation	.20 (.56)	1.53 (3.02)	.00 (.00)	3.31	c<b

a = ADD children groups; b = stuttering children groups; c = general children groups

disfluencies fall into the category of typical disfluencies. In addition, no differential diagnosis of cluttering was presented in the Jang and Shin study. Therefore, this study's results are difficult to interpret regarding stuttering. There may be a cluttering component present in the participating children in this study.

The ability of people with ADD to adjust their speech rate to the linguistic complexity of the utterance determines whether they also exhibit cluttering. Assessment of speech in different speech conditions, with and without medications, is necessary to confirm or reject a cluttering diagnosis. The effect of AD(H)D medications on speech production is an essential aspect to consider as well. Medications such as Ritalin inhibit hyperactive behaviors in general and may reduce the speech rate resulting in the decrease of cluttering symptoms.

5.1.6 Neurogenic cluttering and dysarthria

Cluttering that develops in adulthood because of a neurological disorder is called neurogenic cluttering. The symptoms observed in neurogenic cluttering usually are manifested after brain damage or disease caused by impairment to the basal ganglia system, as is also the case with Parkinson's disease (Alm, 2011). Parkinson's disease results from the death of nerve cells in the substantia nigra and the loss of dopamine and melanin produced by those cells. Dopamine is needed as a "messenger" in the brain, which allows different nerve cells to communicate with each other. If this process is disrupted, problems in motor skills arise, such as problems with walking, dressing, talking,

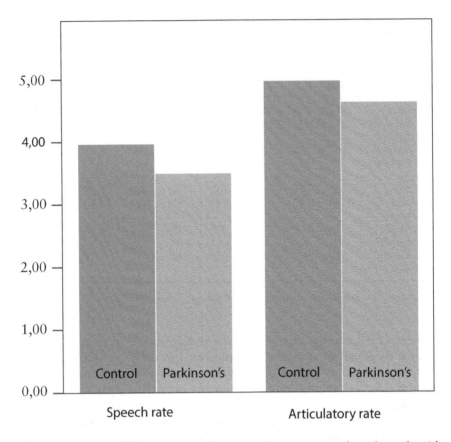

Figure 5.1 Ratio of speech and articulatory rate between controls and people with
         Parkinson's disease

or eating (limited or slow movements), tremors of the arms and sometimes
also the legs, increased muscle tension (stiffness), and difficulty maintaining
balance and falling (Parkinson NL z.j.). The disease spreads to other parts
of the basal ganglia (see Chapter 1, Section 1.4) and to the nerves that control the muscles, involving other neurotransmitters. The main characteristic
of people with neurogenic cluttering is their fast speech rate (De Nil et al.,
2007; Van Borsel & Tetnowski, 2007). Baumgartner (1999) introduced some
speech tasks to differentiate between cluttering and other neurogenic fluency
disorders. Although the disfluencies of PWC are more variable than those of
people with neurogenic fluency disorders, an exacerbation of symptoms in
simple speech tasks is a sign of a neurogenic disorder.

   In the literature, some cases of neurogenic cluttering are described in relation to people who, in addition to multiple sclerosis (MS) or Parkinson's disease also experience cluttering-like symptoms. MS is a central nervous system
disease, inflammation occurs in the brain and spinal cord, which damages

the insulating layer of the nerve (myelin), so nerve signals can no longer be adequately transmitted. In MS, slurred speech is related to losing control over the mouth and muscles of the vocal cords, which become stiffer, and to changing sensations in the mouth and tongue. MS has many symptoms, of which slurred speech (dysarthria) is the symptom that affects communication the most. Terband et al. (2013) studied the similarities between the speech production of individuals with Parkinson's disease and individuals with phonological cluttering. Stable mandibular movements were described as a stable movement pattern, amplitude, and duration (Hartinger & Mooshammer, 2008). In addition, it has been noted that stable jaw movement positively influences speech intelligibility (Smith et al., 1995). This study revealed that jaw movements in the coronal plane of people with Parkinson's disease are significantly more static than such movements in controls and are similar to those of individuals with cluttering. These results suggest that assessing lateral movement stability is important for speech disorder identification and may provide initial direction for intervention planning.

Patients with Parkinson's disease present with a characteristic pattern of impaired speech rhythm. A study conducted by Martínez-Sánchez et al. (2016) reveals that disfluencies in Parkinson's disease result from movement disorders that affect the physiology of the speech production system.

Multiple studies have been done on the speech rate in individuals with Parkinson's disease. A recent study by Martínez-Sánchez et al. (2016) assessed the speech rate, the articulatory rate, and the pause duration in both linguistically correct and incorrect locations. Based on this study, it is clear that the articulatory rate is higher than the speech rate in individuals with Parkinson's Disease and in controls (see also Figure 5.1). This is caused primarily by

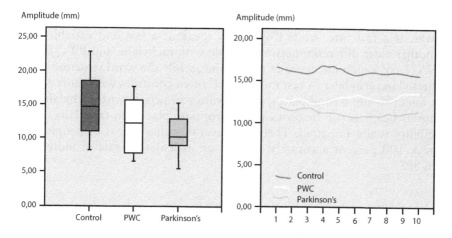

Figure 5.2 Amplitude of jaw movement. Controls (dark gray), PWC (white), individuals with Parkinson's disease (light gray). Left at group level and right per individual

many additional pauses. It is also clear that the mean articulatory rate of individuals with Parkinson's Disease is comparable to that of normal speakers. However, as with cluttering, the excessive number of typical disfluencies and/or the moments of reduced intelligibility give the impression that the speech rate is considerably faster than the speech rate obtained by objective measurements in people with Parkinson's disease.

Van Zaalen and Van Wanseele (2012) concluded that moderate temporal variability with high spatial variability – in other words, flexibility – in jaw movement is essential for normal speech intelligibility (see Figure 5.2). Furthermore, both PWC and people with Parkinson's showed fewer jaw openings than fluent speakers. In other words, the accurate but limited jaw opening during speech production of PWC and people with Parkinson's disease has a negative effect on their intelligibility. However, the reason for this limited jaw movement is probably different for each condition.

5.2   Cluttering and other forms of speech rate that are excessively fast or excessively slow

This section will discuss the disorders known for their excessively fast or slow pace: tachylalia (Section 5.2.1); NF1 (5.2.2); fragile X syndrome (5.2.3); Down syndrome (5.2.4); specific learning difficulties (5.2.5); childhood apraxia of speech (5.2.6); and Tourette's syndrome (5.2.7).

5.2.1   *Cluttering and tachylalia*

Tachylalia is characterized by a fast speech rate without neurological symptoms or psychological etiology. Tachylalia and cluttering can be easily differentiated. In the fast speech rate of a person with tachylalia, speech fluency and syllable structure remain intact. People with tachylalia always speak at a fast rate, while PWC often speak at a fast and variable rate. Another clear difference between people with tachylalia and PWC is that PWC have a high incidence of telescoping, while the word structure is not affected in tachylalia. A fast rate in PWC often coincides with short pauses in linguistically wrong places, while pauses in people with tachylalia are shorter but occur in linguistically appropriate places. In tachylalia, intelligibility is not impaired. There are several online videos of people who speak 100 percent accurately, even at an articulatory rate of more than ten SPS.

5.2.2   *Cluttering and neurofibromatosis type 1*

Cosyns et al. (2012) conducted a study on the articulatory skills of 43 Flemish NF1 patients (14 children and 29 adults), ranging in age between seven and 53 years, in which speech samples were collected using a standardized speech test where all Flemish single speech sounds and most consonant clusters occur in all their allowable syllable positions. The study found that more

Rate of speech	Condition	Speech characteristics	Underlying causes
Too fast or too slow	Gilles de la Tourette syndrome	• High frequency of typical disfluencies in medial and final positions	• Tics • Possibly due to abnormal dopamine levels
	Dyspraxia of speech	• No speech rate adjustment • Inconsistent phonological errors	• Motor speech disorder
	Intellectual disabilities	• typical disfluencies • problems in story structure • grammatical errors • reduced vocabulary	• A variety of causes
	Down syndrome	• Disfluencies increase with age • Phonetic and phonological problems • Lexical retrieval problems	• 47 chromosomes • Different physical and cognitive development • Dyssynchrony between speech rate and language skills
	Fragile X syndrome	• Fast, incoherent speech • Short emotional outbursts • Difficulty maintaining a topic	• Hereditary • Cognitive deficit • Behavioral and physical characteristics
	Neurofibromatosis Type1	• Fast speech rate • Long speech pauses • Phonetic errors	• Mutations in the NF1 gene • Benign tumors on the skin
Fast and/or irregular	Pure cluttering	• High frequency of typical disfluencies or coarticulation errors	• Rate is not adjusted • Disinhibition of signals in the basal ganglia
Irregular	Tachylalia	• Fast speech rate	• Not a disorder
	Neurogenic cluttering	• Speech motor control disrupted • Over-coarticulation • Fast and unintelligible speech	• Trauma or illness • Problems of the central nervous system
	Attention Deficit Hyperactivity Disorder (ADHD)	• Fast speech • High frequency of typical disfluencies, mainly fillers	• Attention deficit • Possible hyperactivity • Inhibition problems
	Autism	• Abnormal speech timing and rhythm	• Neurobiological developmental disorder • Disturbance in information processing • Problems in social communication
	Stuttering	• Sound, syllable, and word repetitions • Prolongations • Blocks	• Dyssynchrony in speech motor control

Figure 5.3 Relationships between underlying mechanisms and symptoms related to an irregular, fast or slow rate

men than women exhibited an incomplete phonetic inventory and that girls tended to make more articulation errors than boys. In children, cluster reduction and final consonant deletion were observed. Children manifested significantly more articulation errors than adults, suggesting that although the articulation skills of NF1 patients evolve positively with age, articulation problems disappear only partially from childhood to adulthood. As such, the articulation errors of NF1 adults can be considered a residual articulation disorder. Therefore, it can be concluded that the speech of NF1 patients is characterized by mild articulation disorder at an age when this is no longer expected.

Another study by Cosyns et al was the first study to digitally measure the mean articulatory rate (MAR) in adults with neurofibromatosis type 1 (NF1). This study indicated that differences between NF1 patients and controls are most significant in the articulatory rate (Cosyns et al., 2013). Although the frequency of disfluencies between groups was similar, NF1 patients demonstrated a higher MAR, and their pauses were longer and more frequent than those of people in a control group. As a result, patients with NF1 had a slower speech rate and a more varied articulatory rate. In addition, Cosyns et al. (2013) found that the disfluency pattern of NF1 patients is more consistent with cluttering patterns than with stuttering patterns.

5.2.3   *Cluttering and fragile-X syndrome*

Fragile-X syndrome (FXS) is an inherited disorder characterized by intellectual disability and certain behavioral and body characteristics. People with FXS often have a relatively long face, large ears, a pronounced chin, and low muscle tone, resulting in joint hypermobility. Gross motor skills and fine motor skills develop more slowly. People with FXS are usually healthy and have an average life expectancy. Boys with FXS are usually fertile, but they often have enlarged testicles. Girls with FXS are also ordinarily fertile. In addition to a mild to severe intellectual disability, people with FXS have numerous other symptoms. They are often shy and/or avoid eye contact. Because of these symptoms, it is often believed that people with FXS have "autistic traits." In addition, language and speech abnormalities occur, such as fast and sometimes incoherent talking. Men with FXS sometimes present with ADHD-like behaviors. FXS is an X-linked neurobiological developmental disorder that occurs in approximately 1:7.000–11.000 individuals. The disorder is caused by excessive generation of CGG 104 trinucleotide. The sequence repeats on the FMR1 gene (Hunter et al., 2014). The FMR1 (fragile X mental retardation 1) gene is responsible for making the protein FMRP (fragile X mental retardation protein), which is essential for cognitive development. FMRP is reduced or absent in FXS (Hagerman et al., 2017). Men are typically more severely affected than women; most men with FXS have an intellectual disability, and approximately 60 percent of them meet the diagnostic criteria for ASD (Bangert et al., 2022). Children with FXS often have symptoms or concomitant diagnoses of anxiety disorders and/or ADHD (Ezell et al., 2019). Speech and language disorders are also common in this population, and impaired speech intelligibility is a prominent characteristic of the FXS communication profile (Bangert et al., 2022).

Children with FXS often manifest rapid bursts of speech and abnormal speech flow, including repetitions of sounds, words, and phrases. The speech of these children is described as compulsive, perseverative, or similar to cluttering. Gillberg (1992) states that cluttering speech is typical for FXS and is not observed in any of the other ASD groups. Poor topic maintenance with frequent unrelated comments may be evidenced. The syntax is usually appropriate for the mental age of people with FXS; they usually show a high receptive vocabulary score; however, their auditory sensory and processing skills are weak (Scharfenaker & Stackhouse, 2012). Boys with FXS, regardless of their autism status, exhibit abnormal phonological characteristics (consonant distortions, with a presence of simplifying phonological processes) like those of younger, normally developing children but are nevertheless less intelligible in connected speech (Barnes et al., 2009). The occurrence of cluttering in people with FXS is disputed by Van Borsel et al. (2008). In their study of the disfluencies in the speech of French-speaking individuals with FXS, Van Borsel et al. (2008) have found a mean speech rate below the norm, indicating that a fast rate is not a consistent characteristic in this population. In response to the finding suggested by Van Borsel et al., it may be suggested that the process of adjusting the rate to the language complexity is much more complicated than just measuring the speech rate. It is much more important to look at the variability and the effect of rate on sentence and word structure (van Zaalen, 2009). As St. Louis et al. (2007) state, and as mentioned several times in this book, the speech rate in cluttering can be perceived as fast, even when the rate, as measured, remains within normal limits.

A comparison study by Zajac et al. (2009) found that boys with FXS and ASD speak significantly faster than their age-matched controls. Multiple linear regression demonstrates that the articulation rate, with the final word of the sentence and with sentence-final fundamental frequency (F0) reduction, accounts for 91 percent of the variance for the observed rate. Zajac et al. (2009) conclude that atypical sentence-final prosody may be attributed to the perceived rate in boys with FXS and ASD.

Cluttering is a disorder that has been clinically observed in individuals with FXS. However, this population needs to be evaluated systematically to confirm the cluttering diagnosis, which is a process necessary for identification and possible intervention. A recent study by Bangert et al. (2022) examines the articulatory rate in young adult males with FXS using expert clinical advice, the alignment between the clinical opinion of experts and objectively quantified characteristics of cluttering from language transcripts, and the association between cluttering and aspects of the FXS phenotype. In total, speech samples from 36 men with FXS (ages 18–26;

M = 22, SD 2.35) were analyzed for nonverbal cognition, autism, anxiety, and ADD symptoms. The consensus of two clinical experts in fluency disorders has determined the presence of cluttering based on characteristics exhibited in the language sample.

Cluttering-like characteristics (speech rate, disfluencies, etc.) were also objectively quantified based on language transcriptions. The study determined that 50 percent of the participants met the criteria for a cluttering diagnosis. Phrase repetitions were the most significant feature that distinguished individuals who presented with cluttering. Although cluttering was not associated with autism symptoms or the mean length of utterance, cluttering was more likely identified when nonverbal cognitive abilities were higher, when ADD symptoms were more evident, and when anxiety symptoms were minimal.

5.2.4   Cluttering and Down syndrome

In 1866, John Langdon Down referred to the speech of people with the syndrome that would later be named after him in terms that are consistent with a diagnosis of cluttering (Van Borsel, 2011). Disfluencies in the speech of adults with intellectual disabilities are usually considered stuttering in the comparison process and patient records, and treatment focuses on stuttering. Notably, very little research has been published to distinguish aspects of disfluency in this specific population (Coppens-Hofman et al., 2013). One recurring issue in the literature in this area is whether the disfluent speech in people with Down syndrome (DS) is characterized by stuttering or cluttering (Van Borsel, 2011).

The underlying causes of speech disfluencies in people with DS are likely to differ from the causes of disfluencies in children without intellectual disabilities. Causes for disfluencies can be attributed to other problems, such as impaired cognitive functioning, limited knowledge of language and vocabulary, poor concentration, memory difficulties, side effects of medications, auditory input problems, and other comorbidities. Eggers and Van Eerdenbrugh (2018) suggest that children with DS have different types of disfluencies compared to normally developing children. One of the few longitudinal studies on fluency and intelligibility in young children with DS, was conducted by Deckers (2015) (see the following theory block).

Children with DS often experience speech problems. Although the exact nature and origin of the speech problems associated with DS have yet to be determined, it is generally accepted that these problems often lead to significantly reduced intelligibility (Kumin, 2006) and problems in speech fluency.

Children's speech errors in DS do not just reflect their delayed language acquisition. More than half of DS children's words are pronounced differently on repeated productions in a picture-naming task (Dodd & Thompson, 2001), whereas typically developing children produce less than 10 percent of the words inconsistently (Burt et al., 1999). Children with delayed phonological development have an inconsistency rating of less than 20 percent (Dodd, 1995). There are different opinions about factors affecting the ability to speak with the precise articulation needed for clear and fluent speech. Speech problems in individuals with DS are often characterized by: (1) a specific physiological and anatomical profile, including a smaller than average oral cavity, hypotonia of muscles around the mouth, fusion of lip muscles, and an excessive amount of lip musculature (Miller et al., 1999), and additional problems in speech motor control; (2) a phonological delay (Chair-Gammon, 2001; Van Borsel, 1996); (3) signs of dyspraxia (Kumin, 2006); and (4) hearing loss (Dodd & Thompson, 2001). The most common characteristics in seven children with DS are reduced intelligibility in longer utterances, inconsistency of speech errors, reduced ability to perform voluntary tasks compared to automatic tasks, and difficulty sequencing oral movements and speech sounds (Kumin & Adams, 2000). In addition to the previously mentioned causal factors in speech problems, intelligibility can also be compromised by speech disfluency. Several studies showed many disfluencies in people with DS, but data on different disfluencies are rarely provided (Bray, 2003; Devenny & Silverman, 1990; Van Borsel & Vandermeulen, 2008). Researchers such as Otto and Yairi (1975) and Coppens-Hofman et al. (2013) focused on differentiating disfluencies. Where Stansfield (1990) concluded that 14 to 77 percent of the total DS population was disfluent, with a ratio of 13 PWS to 2 PWC, Van Borsel and Vandermeulen (2008) reported that 78.9 percent of children with DS were diagnosed with cluttering, and 17.1 percent were classified as combined cases of cluttering and stuttering. Moreover, although the reported rates of fluency problems in children with DS are relatively high, knowledge about their fluency disorders is minimal. There are some reports of stuttering and cluttering-like features in the DS population.

The study by Deckers et al. (2015) used a questionnaire focusing on speech, language, and fluency based on Kumin's (2006) profile. The questionnaire was expanded with questions about speech sound acquisition, fluency, motor performance, phonological coding, and speech rate. With an expert review of speech therapists, physiotherapists, DS specialists, parents, and doctors, the validity of this questionnaire was guaranteed. The questionnaire was completed by 115 parents of children with DS (age 1.0–6.11 years). The children had an average age of 2.10 years (SD 1.6), and the group consisted of 63.5 percent boys. A pilot study with 25 typically developing children and six children with DS indicated a high correlation between parental responses and spontaneous speech analysis, based on the assumption that parents can accurately identify acquired sounds and disfluencies in their children. Cross-sectional results on all factors were analyzed between and within age groups.

Results

Intelligibility scores vary significantly across age groups (see Figure 5.4). Older children with DS tend to have higher intelligibility scores than younger children. In the age groups of 1- and 2-year-olds, a highly positive correlation was found between syllable deletion and speech rate. The intelligibility scores are strongly correlated with the correct production of consonant clusters, especially in the groups of 2-year-old ($r = .467$), 3-year-old ($r = .542$), and 4-year-old ($r = .602$) children with DS.

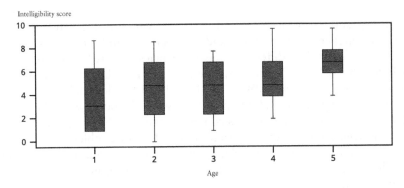

Figure 5.4 Intelligibility scores of children with DS by age group

Fluency development

At age 1, 12.5 percent of DS children manifested stuttering-like disfluencies (prolongations), and 6.3 percent exhibited typical disfluencies. With age, the number of children experiencing fluency problems increases, but 58 percent of DS children in this study have never experienced any fluency disruptions. Typical disfluencies were recorded in 21.6 percent of all cases. A combination of blockages and prolongations was seen in 4.3 percent of all cases. Blockages correlated positively with problems in rhythm ($r = .442$).

Phonological coding problems increase with age and are characterized in the study by syllable deletion, telescoping, and sequencing order (Deckers et al., 2019) (see Table 5.3). The number of distorted consonants in clusters increases with age. It remains to be seen whether this is related to phonetic planning, motor programming problems, or

Table 5.3 Fluency, motor skills, rate, speech, and language development in children with DS by age group (Deckers et al., 2019)

Down Syndrome (N=115)		Age									
		1 (N=16)		2 (N=30)		3 (N=30)		4 (N=14)		5 (N=25)	
		(Almost) always	Not (yet)	(Almost) always	Not (yet)	(Almost) always	Not (yet)	(Almost) always	Not (yet)	(Almost) always	Not (yet)
Fluency	Blocks	0.0	100	0.0	100	16.7	83.3	28.6	71.4	16.0	84.0
	Repetitions	6.3	93.8	16.7	83.3	26.7	73.3	28.6	71.4	24.0	76.0
	Prolongations	12.5	87.5	30.0	70.0	26.7	73.3	28.6	71.4	8.0	92.0
Motor	Facial muscle tension	0.0	100	6.7	93.3	16.7	83.3	14.3	85.7	4.0	96.0
	Singing	0.0	100	3.3	96.7	13.3	86.7	21.4	78.6	12.0	88.0
	Rhythm variation	0.0	100	0.0	100	10.0	90.0	14.3	85.7	12.0	88.0
Rate	Fast rate	6.3	93.8	3.3	96.7	10.0	90.0	28.6	71.4	12.0	88.0
Speech	Clusters problems	0.0	100	6.7	93.3	23.3	76.7	35.7	64.3	60.0	40.0
	Syllable deletion	12.5	87.5	20.0	80.0	30.0	70.0	35.7	64.3	32.0	68.0
	Telescoping	0.0	100	6.7	93.3	26.7	73.3	21.4	78.6	36.0	64.0
	Sequencing	0.0	100	3.3	96.7	23.3	76.7	28.6	71.4	28.0	72.0
	Word > sentences	6.3	93.8	33.3	66.7	36.7	63.3	28.6	71.4	32.0	68.0
	Longer words	12.5	87.5	36.7	63.3	56.7	43.3	50.0	50.0	44.0	56.0
Language	Plural	0.0	100	3.3	96.7	10.0	90.0	14.3	85.7	40.0	60.0
	Past tense	0.0	100	0.0	100.0	0.0	100.0	7.1	92.9	16.0	84.0

environmental circumstances. Motor execution problems manifested by weak facial muscle tone during singing seem to occur less frequently after the age of 5 years.

Significant, but medium or low, correlations were found between age and intelligibility (r = .265); correct production of consonant clusters (r = .484); morphological markers, such as plural (r = .387) and past tense (r = .283); blocks (r = .240); and vocals (r = .172). No high correlations (r > .5) were found between age and other variables, indicating non-age-dependent development in children with Down syndrome.

Summary

Although all children with DS experience language difficulties, especially in expressive language skills, the development of the most basic neurocognitive and perceptual processes related to communication competence differs from child to child. Different individuals, therefore, need different skills to achieve communicative competence (Light, 1997). Thus, a comprehensive assessment of linguistic functioning is needed. In this study, linguistic performance in the DS group was significantly reduced at both semantic and phonological levels.

As Nash and Snowling (2008) suggested, the differences in speech-language and fluency development in children with DS may reflect less efficient retrieval strategies, rather than differences in the organization of linguistic representations. Speech patterns in DS are a combination of delayed language acquisition and errors not observed in normal development. Delayed developmental patterns and abnormal non-developmental patterns are evident at the approximate age of three years. Together, the findings pointed to the need to control DS deficits rather than impaired language processes. Disfluencies in the DS population in this study indicated a distribution as seen in the general population and not a high frequency of stuttering-like disfluencies. Disfluencies in this DS population were therefore considered an indication of dyssynchrony, as introduced by Myers (1992), between the speech-language system and the rate of execution. Answers on parental questionnaires based on descriptions of symptoms that may or may not be present in the child's communication provided more insight into fluency development compared to diagnosis-based questionnaires (as used in studies in the twentieth century).

The parental questionnaires used in previous studies asked parents whether their children had stuttering or another fluency problem. Parents were not given a precise definition of these phenomena or asked about the frequency or type of disfluencies or their severity. Extensive longitudinal research regarding DS children has not been reported, except for the study by Deckers et al. (2015).

5.2.5 Cluttering and specific learning difficulties

Tiger et al. (1980) investigated similarities between cluttering and specific learning disabilities. Daly (1992) also noted such similarities, pointing out that many symptoms experienced by PWC are also present in people with learning difficulties or learning disabilities. Daly referred to symptoms such as impulsivity, lack of order and awareness, inattention, underachievement at school, specific reading difficulties, and language disorders. According to Daly (1992) and Mensink-Ypma (1990), additional common difficulties for PWC and individuals with learning difficulties are problems with writing and dysrhythmic speech. Although the symptoms are similar, the underlying processes that result in the symptoms of both conditions are different, and the rate of improvement can vary.

Because there are problems in the language formulation in PWC and people with specific learning disabilities, Preus (1996) concluded that cluttering has more in common with people with learning disabilities than with PWS. This idea was previously suggested by Mensink-Ypma (1990). All of the above-mentioned characteristics are based on clinical observations by speech therapists. They are described in relatively vague terms, such as "difficulties in the formulation of language" or "unawareness of speech symptoms." Recent research shows differences in type, severity, and underlying processes in the language performance of PWC and people with learning disabilities. The differences in speech and language characteristics of these two populations are described below.

In a Dutch study (N = 150; age 10.6–12.11 years), Van Zaalen et al. (2009d) found that adolescents with cluttering scored similarly in terms of their articulation rate as people with learning disabilities. Children with cluttering differ from children with learning disabilities by:

1. a higher frequency of typical disfluencies;
2. a higher number of semantic paraphasia;
3. the presence of grammatical errors in speech but not in writing;
4. a higher percentage of main issues, side issues, and noise while narrating a story;
5. more problems with story structure.

We will now discuss the differences in speech and language production between PWC and people with learning disabilities.

1 A higher frequency of typical disfluencies

The typical disfluencies of PWC consist mainly of word and sentence repetitions. PWC may use them to gain time to convert their thoughts into speech in order to gain time for speech planning and execution. Children with learning disabilities use primarily interjections, such as "um," to buy time for lexical retrieval. In addition, planning an idea or a message is difficult for this group. In addition to their typical disfluencies, people with learning disabilities produce disfluencies that are not typical and cannot be categorized as stuttering-like or normal disfluencies; for example, repetitions of the final syllable of words (Coppens-Hofman et al., 2013).

2   *A higher number of semantic paraphasias*

PWC use semantically related words and phonological paraphasias. In the latter, a speaker constructs a word with a high degree of phonological similarities; he says, for example, "I choose a fruit," when "I choose a flight" was meant. After production, these errors are not corrected but are only detected by the speaker when a recording is played back. Children with learning disabilities frequently use semantic paraphasia quite often. When making these kinds of mistakes, PWC have the right concept in mind and want to express it, but eventually, a sentence with a different meaning is inadvertently produced. Tatyana, a person with cluttering, recalled, for example: "I also had to learn how to overcome the desire to never open my mouth again after producing sentences in a disjointed story . . ." (Exum et al., 2010). PWC fail to retrieve the correct word from their lexicon and are unaware of that error unless it is pointed out to them. They do notice the error when a recording is played back repeatedly. For example, Charlene described such an experience as follows: "The competition usually resulted in a jumbled mass of words exiting my mouth, leaving both recipient and myself perplexed" (Exum et al., 2010).

3   *Making grammatical errors in speech, but not when writing*

Errors in sentence structure in cluttering only occur in spoken language, not in written language. PWC do not make grammatical errors when they are able to focus sufficiently on their speech. People with learning disabilities, however, make grammatical errors in both written and spoken language.

4   *Normal usage of main issues, side issues, and noise*

Research by Van Zaalen et al. (2009) suggested that children with learning disabilities produced fewer main and secondary issues and an excessive amount of noise, such as the interjections "I don't remember it" or "What did you say again?" or additional sentences that were not originally in the story. PWC tend to use main and side issues as frequently as fluent speakers, but they also produce an excessive amount of noise.

5   *Few errors in story sequence*

Children with learning disabilities have major problems retelling stories in sequence. When retelling stories, they make errors in the sequence of story elements without awareness (for example: "My father drives to Amsterdam and sat in the car"). PWC do not notice such narrative structure errors in their speech. Moreover, stories told by PWC can be perceived as chaotic due to the high frequency of disfluencies and telescoping combined with a fast speech rate and frequent instances of noise. Their story structure is usually accurate.

5.2.6   *Cluttering in developmental apraxia of speech*

Developmental apraxia of speech (DAS) is a disorder in which the coordination of sequenced speech movements is disturbed. DAS refers to an inconsistent ability to perform specific targeted motor movements. These are problems in the planning and coordination of muscle movements. The distinctive feature of DAS is that people with this condition cannot make certain movements intentionally but can only make them involuntarily, while unaware of them. For example, children with DAS can blow into their teacup when it is too hot but may have difficulty producing the /f/ phoneme in isolation.

Nijland (2009) assumes that there is a problem in syllable planning in children with DAS. Their speech is less stable than necessary for effortless and error-free speech production and thus becomes insufficiently automated. Errors similar to those made by children with DAS are sometimes made by PWC, such as sound distortions, indicating abnormal synchronization of articulatory sequencing, and serial order in the speech of PWC (Ward, 2011). Although DAS and cluttering have different etiologies, these disorders have noticeable similarities. We discuss the similarities first before discussing the differences in Table 5.4:

- The adjustment of the speech rate differs according to speaking conditions.
- The speech rate of children with DAS and PWC does not adjust to different speech conditions, although in DAS, the speech rate is often slow, while in cluttering, the speech rate is often fast (Dannenbauer, 1999).
- People with apraxia often search for the appropriate articulation placement by producing groping movements of the mouth, a phenomenon known as SOD. However, in cluttering such movements can occur only when the speech rate is too fast.
- The variability of repeated production in multisyllabic words differs: People with DAS and PWC show high variability in repeated productions of the same word; for people with DAS, this happens in both low- and high-frequency words, while only the low-frequency words are affected in PWC.
- The frequent deletion of terminal consonants: Deletion of final consonants can occur in people with DAS, as well as in PWC.
- Additions of sounds: Additions of sounds can hinder the speech intelligibility of children with DAS. In cluttering, sounds are added when the speech rate is too fast or when complex multisyllabic words are used.

Table 5.4 Characteristics of cluttering and DAS (Van Zaalen & Winkelman, 2014)

Characteristic	Cluttering	DAS
Age when most symptoms can be identified	Pre-adolescence	Toddlers
Variability of productions	High	High
Speech rate	High	Low
Searching mouth movements	Yes, but only at a fast speech rate	Yes
Initial sound substitutions	None	Possible
Deletion of final consonants	Possible	Possible
Addition of sound(s)	Yes, at a fast rate	Yes

5.2.7 Tourette's syndrome (TS)

No research has been published on cluttering in relation to Tourette's syndrome (TS). The putamen, which is a part of the basal ganglia, appears to be involved in coordinating automatic behaviors, such as riding a bicycle or driving. Therefore, problems with the putamen can explain the symptoms of TS. The most apparent reason for the lack of research on cluttering and TS is that TS may be related to the extrapyramidal motor system, which causes abnormal reflexes and involuntary movements. In contrast, this extrapyramidal motor system is not known to be impaired in PWC. De Nil et al. (2005) analyzed the fluency of 69 children with TS while reading and in spontaneous speech. They found that children with TS had an overall higher frequency of more typical (or normal) disfluencies compared to controls. In contrast to stuttering-like and typical disfluencies, disfluencies of children with TS occurred primarily in the medial and final word positions.

These findings are supported by a study conducted by Van Borsel and Vanryckeghem (2000), who noted that interjections were the predominant type of disfluency in people with TS. Interjections accounted for 48.2 percent of all disfluencies that were identified in a case study of an 18-year-old man with TS. Cluttering in people with TS is characterized primarily by a significant number of typical disfluencies, such as sentence and word repetitions, interjections, frequent revisions, and incomplete sentences, resulting in disorganized linguistic output (Van Borsel, 2011).

Speech therapists should thoroughly investigate whether inhibition of motor activity occurs in their TS patients. A potentially useful tool would be to create questionnaires about atypical tics to collect information about their prevalence, duration, age of onset, and correlation with other tics. The use of such a tool in daily practice could make it possible to diagnose more patients correctly, and it will facilitate further research (Kaczynska & Janik, 2021).

5.3 Reliability of existing data in relation to cluttering and other disorders, diseases, and syndromes

There are many factors that play a role in the diagnosis of cluttering, both in clinical practice and in scientific research. These factors are the definition (section 5.3.1), the language complexity (5.3.2), and the coexisting conditions.

5.3.1 Symptoms of cluttering are not accounted for

The definition of St. Louis et al. (2011) provides three clear symptoms of cluttering, which are recognized by experts worldwide. Reduced attention to the process of speaking is not viewed as a pivotal consideration in this definition, while – as will be discussed in Chapters 6 and 7 –this aspect is of great importance, both for the assessment and for the treatment of cluttering.

40-second rule

Experience shows that PWC are unable to adjust their speech rate to the linguistic demands of the moment for more than 30 to 40 seconds. After that, their uncontrolled automatic speech returns.

Diagnoses of the disorders and syndromes described above often depend on the number of disfluencies. However, disfluencies are usually mentioned as a single variable, with no information provided about the speech rate and how these disfluencies influence intelligibility, etc. As a result, typical disfluencies continue to be erroneously identified by various researchers as stuttering-like disfluencies. This applies, for example, to word repetitions with less than three iterations. Such disfluencies are more common in fluent speech. Differential diagnostic characteristics, such as frequency variation or sentence and word structures, are rarely considered during diagnostic evaluations.

5.3.2 The influence of language complexity

Not referring to cluttering as a language disorder in St. Louis' definition of cluttering is more complex, especially since the symptoms such as the high number of typical disfluencies indicate problems in the word finding or grammatical coding and errors in the word structure indicate problems in phonological coding (Bretherton-Furness & Ward, 2012; Van Zaalen & Reichel, 2015, 2019; Van Zaalen et al., 2009, 2009b; Van Zaalen & Dejonckere, 2010).

The definition of St. Louis et al. (2011) is considered the LCD definition. It was intended to limit the number of symptoms to the minimum to be acceptable to most international scientific community members. This definition allows researchers to succeed in the empirical and clinical exploration of cluttering for many years. Yet, one significant factor related to the causes of cluttering must be clarified. The definition of St. Louis et al. (2011) does not refer to cluttering as a disorder of language. One of the symptoms of cluttering identified in this definition is an excessive number of normal dysfluencies. People manifest such a high number of normal dysfluencies because of word-finding or difficulties in grammatical encoding. Another symptom in the definition of St. Louis et al. (2011) is telescoping, which is a problem in word structure, indicating a deficit in phonological encoding. Therefore, some of the symptoms identified by the definition of St. Louis et al. (2011) are caused by the impaired encoding of language in PWC. This factor is consistent with and expanded in the definition of van Zaalen and Reichel (2022). Their causative definition of cluttering not only includes the mandatory symptoms of the definition of St. Louis et al. (2011), but also explains the correlation between the abnormal adjustment of the articulatory rate to the demands of all language components at the moment of speech, and specifies which components of language are affected in syntactic and phonological types of cluttering, respectively.

What is unique to cluttering is that the symptoms occur only in a higher level of language complexity contexts if the rate of speech is too fast to retrieve the necessary words and/or encode complex sentence constructions. In contexts with lower levels of language complexity, the frequency of typical disfluencies is similar to that of typical speakers This difference can even be observed by comparing the number of disfluencies in retelling a story by the PWC with the number of disfluencies in retelling a story.

Further research using the current definitions of cluttering in the aforementioned disorders, considering fluency, rate, phonology, and intelligibility in various conversational contexts—especially in connected speech samples—is necessary to adequately promote our knowledge of disfluencies and intelligibility in these subgroups (St. Louis et al., 2007; Van Zaalen, 2009).

5.4   Conclusion

In summary, this chapter covers cluttering characteristics, analyses of cluttering symptoms, and interpretations of a variety of empirical studies, which will provide an understanding of the initial differential diagnosis of cluttering and related disorders. Comprehensive and accurate tools are proposed for differentiating between cluttering and various other conditions with common characteristics and secondary symptoms.

Part 3
Therapy

6   Therapeutic considerations

6.1   Therapy plan

A therapy plan can be formulated after a client with cluttering describes their problem, based on the results of Predictive Cluttering Inventory-revised (PCI-r) (See Chapter 3, Section 3.1) and the Brief Cluttering and Stuttering Questionnaire (BCSQ) (see Chapter 4, Section 4.8). In addition, the assessment should include the Cluttering Assessment Battery (CAB) in conjunction with diagnostic exercises. Data obtained by taking the history and evaluating the assessment results should provide sufficient information on specific symptoms of cluttering for each client. Reducing or managing these symptoms is the goal of cluttering therapy.

After the assessment, the intervention should be planned and tailored to each client. The prognosis for the client should be based on the type, number, and severity of the symptoms that need to be addressed. In addition, the client's ability to learn and change contributes to the therapy outcome. Lastly, a comprehensive assessment of the client provides insights into approaches to cluttering intervention, including therapeutic methods, types of exercises, and audio-visual resources.

This chapter provides an overview of general considerations for cluttering therapy, such as changes in social communication, problems in the monitoring of speech, the four-component model of Stourneras (1980) and cluttering therapy, priorities in the treatment of people with cluttering and stuttering, exercise hierarchy, and the intensity of treatment. Then, the impact of cluttering therapy on each client is analyzed in relation to the short- and long-term results. The short-term results can be seen as the immediate impact on speaking behavior, cognitions, and emotions. Achieving long-term results in the treatment of cluttering is challenging; therefore, results can only be achieved through short periods of intensive training within communicative contexts.

Stourneras' (1980) four-component model, consisting of cognitive, emotional, verbal-motor, and communicative components, will be explained in terms of how clients can be helped to improve their performance in all four of these components. The chapter presents therapeutic considerations related to issues such as planning the client-focused intervention, and daily practice

DOI: 10.4324/9781003460558-9

with exercises aimed at improving speech, identification of symptoms, attention skills, and memory. Special attention is paid to facilitating expressive and receptive language skills and increasing organizational, pragmatic, lexical, and conversational skills. A discussion of the hierarchy of the exercises and the intensity of the treatment is also included.

6.2   Impact of therapy

Cluttering therapy involves more than changing the speech of PWC. It creates transformations in many areas of communication that transcend routine speaking exercises. Such work includes training targeted speech, formulating the message, and developing a different listening attitude or focus on a partner. PWC that have poor speech intelligibility may not be able to interpret the listeners' feedback accurately. The following example illustrates how a person with cluttering could not correctly read cues of a listener's response to her speech.

> Anouschka, a 23-year-old geography student, says: "I was in a bar two weeks ago with a friend I hadn't seen in a long time. I drank two beers, and we had a very lively conversation. I had a wonderful evening. Then, a few days ago, I saw my friend again. She said to me, 'Wow, you were so drunk! I couldn't understand a word of what you were saying. Wasn't that fun?' I was stunned. My world collapsed. I really thought she understood me while we were talking, and I wasn't drunk at all."

6.2.1   Transfer and stabilization

Limitations in the ability to produce intelligible and natural speech are caused by various neurological abnormalities and are known to negatively affect the quality of life (Stipancic et al., 2021). Although therapies are available for improving the intelligibility and quality of speech, current interventions have limited effectiveness and often do not result in full recovery of intelligible and natural-sounding speech (Stipancic et al., 2021).

In cluttering therapy, a client's effort in performing an exercise is considered positive (intrinsic reward). Once a client is better understood, they find their communication pleasant again. This positive change yields immediate, encouraging results. Due to the slow development of the internal feedback loop for the clients, the danger of a relapse is an immediate concern. This is why it is important to schedule therapy sessions frequently in the beginning (daily practice by the client and weekly feedback by the therapist). Because cluttering does not disappear but becomes manageable, it is important to gradually reduce the therapy frequency in the monitoring phase. This offers the best opportunities to facilitate maintenance and stabilization. Relapse can be prevented by a client increasing their self-management skills, particularly in monitoring and adjusting their speaking behavior. The term "transfer" refers to the application of learned skills in daily communication and in life in general. Effective transfer increases the chance of stabilization.

Stabilization refers to the learned skills which have become fully automatic without a high probability of relapse. In such a situation, the client can monitor their speech by agreeing with people close to them to provide feedback about their speech and/or by regular self-evaluation of their speech, supported by PRAAT speech analysis software.

> Rapid speech cannot be changed, but it can be effectively monitored!

When a client has improved their skills and achieved their goals in various speaking situations, they should focus on preventing relapses. It is, therefore, important to carry out regular follow-up evaluations, preferably by the client themselves. Regular follow-up evaluations can also be carried out by scheduling appointments with the speech therapist at appropriate times or by sending clients' recordings to the speech therapist for analysis via e-mail at regular intervals. The frequency of such follow-up evaluations should decrease over time. The client must have various tools to practice their newly acquired speech behavior efficiently. The most effective approach is to use audio-visual feedback (AVF) training with recorded conversations (see Chapter 7, Section 7.4).

Speech therapists can advise clients with cluttering to evaluate new gains the day after they are achieved. If therapy does not yield satisfactory results within a week, PWC should be advised to restart their training independently. If these additional training sessions do not yield satisfactory results within two weeks, the PWC should get in touch with the speech therapist. The generalization of acquired skills starts with the first session by practicing within a specific communicative context and should be continued after therapy concludes, ideally for up to two years.

6.2.2 Short- and long-term impact

The short-term results of cluttering treatment are driven by two main factors: a positive change in speech behavior and a positive effect on cognitions and emotions. The effect on speech behavior can be significant, especially when a client is able to apply new behavior in other situations (transfer) and manage to stabilize newly improved speech behavior. Achieving long-term results within a treatment is challenging when the treatment is carried out at a low intensity and without objective measurements. To achieve SMART goals (See Section 6.7), short periods of intense training are recommended (ten to twelve weeks per goal).

AVF training appears to be effective treatment for cluttering

In 2019, Van Zaalen and Reichel published the results of a study on the effectiveness of training with audio-visual feedback (AVF) on PWC regarding articulatory accuracy, pause duration, frequency and type of disfluencies, as well as the emotional and cognitive aspects that may be typical for PWC. In their study, 12 male adolescents and adults — six with phonological and six with syntactic cluttering — received weekly AVF training over a 12-week period, with a follow-up after three months. Data was collected at baseline (T0), week 6 (T1), week 12 (T2), and after follow-up (T3). In addition, the spontaneous speech was recorded and analyzed using the digital audio recording and speech analysis software PRAAT (Boersma & Weenink, 2019, 2022).

In the above-mentioned study, PWC showed significant improvements in their articulatory rate and pause duration after the AVF training. In addition, the PWC reported positive effects on their ability to retell a story and speak in more complete sentences. The PWC felt better at formulating their ideas and were more satisfied with their interactions with those around them. The AVF training proved to be a sustainable and effective approach to improving the PWC's monitoring skills with both quantitative and qualitative benefits in the behavioral, cognitive, emotional, and social domains of communication. Follow-up research is needed to confirm these results.

Van Zaalen and Reichel (2014) presented a variety of treatment approaches based on an understanding of four components of communication, and describe cluttering therapy aimed at:

- problem identification;
- reduction of speech rate;
- facilitating appropriate pauses;
- facilitating appropriate monitoring.

In addition to therapeutic considerations, and understanding the specifics of cluttering, it is also important to pay close attention to:

- building trust in the clinician;
- the clinician's emotional competencies;
- the sense of accomplishment of PWC;
- converting the therapeutic process into realistic expectations;
- motivating the client to pursue challenging goals;
- strengthening the self-management of PWC.

Since PWC themselves are often not bothered by their cluttering but are frustrated by the reactions of listeners, their experiencing success in the short term is essential for keeping them motivated. Moreover, success in therapy also encourages PWC to monitor their speech and to increase their change readiness (See Chapter 4, Section 4.4).

6.2.3 Impact of cluttering on social communication

Because PWC are unaware of the reasons for their communication problems, they often try to adjust their communication pattern and social behavior to convey their message.

Intuitive adjustment

Eva, a 17-year-old girl, always enters the most critical points and appointments in an email after a telephone conversation where she has discussed or agreed to something. As a result, her colleagues and family have insentiently learned to trust Eva's emails if they did not fully understand her verbal conversation, and they respond via e-mail in case of uncertainty. They feel they do not need to ask Eva for clarification or repetition as often as in the past.

PWC often avoid difficult speaking situations. This avoidance frequently occurs when PWC are unaware that their disfluencies or poor intelligibility is the main reason for the avoidance behavior.

In therapy, it is crucial to work on improving the social interactions of PWC. The Speech Situation Checklist can be used to ascertain which situations should be given the highest priority. Keep in mind that changes in priority can be made over time, due to the success of treatment or a better understanding of the symptoms of clients. Situations that previously seemed

Avoidance behavior in a person with cluttering

Frederik, a 35-year-old curriculum developer at a university, is working with seven of his colleagues on a new curriculum for first-year students. During meetings, Frederik proposes several creative solutions and ideas. His colleagues in the team smile at him but do not respond to the content of his suggestions. Finally, when another colleague in the same team introduces almost identical ideas, this colleague is praised for his inventive spirit, and his ideas are incorporated into the curriculum plan. After this has happened several times, Frederik becomes the team's secretary and no longer shares his thoughts with the team. Although this is a short-term solution (he no longer experiences disappointment), Frederik begins to doubt his value to the team after some time, knowing that he cannot express himself adequately. Two months later, he decides to go for speech and language evaluation and therapy. One of the first goals in therapy is to train Frederik to speak and respond in a targeted manner during team meetings. Upon implementing the lessons, he learned in his therapy, he surprises his colleagues with his knowledge and creativity. As a result, Frederik gives up his role as secretary and rejoins the brainstorming team.

to deserve less priority may become of great importance to the PWC, with time. Although the Speech Situation Checklist is extensive, it is certainly conceivable that there are social contexts that do not appear in the list. Speech therapists need to create a hierarchy of social contexts for their clients and their families.

6.3   Problems in monitoring

As mentioned earlier, the main feature of cluttering is an uncontrollably fast and/or irregular speech rate, which leads, firstly, to problems in the planning and execution of the verbal-motor and linguistic structures, and, secondly, to an inability to accurately monitor language output. When errors are detected, PWC may experience problems making corrections due to their fast speech rate and their very short pauses. Typical speakers recognize slips of the tongue or incorrect sentence formulations due to the so-called internal feedback loop, which is indiscernible to the listener (internal monitoring). Speakers are aware of the quality of their speech and will improve it if necessary. Many slips of the tongue and phrasing errors in speakers that do not clutter are recognized before the utterance is entirely produced. An example of overt monitoring (revision) is: "I've gone home . . . cycled." Sometimes these problems are corrected after producing the whole statement; for example: "I walked home – no, cycled." Although discussed in the literature, there is no conclusive evidence that PWC have monitoring problems in fast speech. However, clinical experience has made it clear that PWC have a limited ability to control their speech when performing complex language tasks. At the same time, there is no doubt that PWC can adequately monitor their speech at a low level of language complexity (for example, reading aloud and counting from one to ten). The inability of PWC to adjust their speech rate to the complexity of the linguistic task detracts from their ability to monitor their speech and language output adequately due to extreme dissynchronicity. This is called a double deficit (Van Zaalen, 2009).

Double deficit in cluttering

Deficiency 1: PWC cannot adequately adjust the rate of speech production, making them disfluent or less intelligible.
  Deficiency 2: PWC cannot adequately monitor their speech, preventing "errors" from being noticed and corrected.

Van Zaalen et al. (2009c)

The level of language complexity at which cluttering symptoms occur and a person's ability to be trained determine the prognosis for the effectiveness of cluttering therapy. Development of monitoring skills at different levels of language complexity is the priority in cluttering therapy. Such therapy begins with the monitoring of language production. The speaker listens to part of the message and compares it with linguistic rules and the intended content of the message. At this level of monitoring, PWC can benefit from auditory, visual, and sensory identification of symptoms. Getting PWC to listen to their own recorded speech is an excellent way to make them aware of their speaking patterns. This can be supported by visual information. Chapter 2, Section 2.2.6 and Chapter 7, Section 7.5 provide examples of visual information generated by the PRAAT software.

6.4 Cluttering's four-component model

Stourneras' four-component model (1980) includes cognitive, emotional, verbal-motor, and communicative components. PWC make every effort for improvement in all four components. In therapy, therefore, attention should be paid not only to the verbal-motor and communicative components but also to the cognitive and emotional components.

6.4.1   *The cognitive component*

Experience shows that PWC fall within a broad continuum of self-awareness and emotional response to their cluttering. These range from denials to incessant worry, and from frustration due to personal speaking deficits to frustration with others' inability to keep up with their rate of speech. PWC may have low communicative self-esteem and may feel misunderstood and incompetent (Reichel, 2010).

> ### A low communicative self-image
>
> Two cluttering teachers were concerned about their students' inability to understand them.
>
> Anouk, who is a speech therapy graduate student who also has cluttering, was worried about his future employment.
>
> Tim, a car mechanic, was saddened by his loss of customers because of his unclear speech.
>
> John-William, a high school student, was annoyed by listeners' frequent requests for them to repeat what they said. This young man attributed all their communication problems to stuttering, despite their speech being notably rapid and difficult to understand due to cluttering.
>
> Nick, another high school student, was frustrated with their poor grades and constant conflict with their peers, because of their poor social control.
>
> Alex, a 13-year-old boy, became despondent because of their mother's insistence that they should do their speech exercises instead of playing video games.

The cognitive component of Stourneras' four-component model has two subcomponents: attention and habituation.

Attention

Every person has a specific capacity for attention, which can be used to focus more intently on tasks. If the language production is automatic, the speaker will use little attention capacity for language production. On the other hand, for a person who speaks very fast and tries to slow down, part of the attention capacity will have to be used to monitor the slowing down of the speech rate. The following example illustrates this process:

Driving a Ferrari

Desirée typically drives a middle-class car to work through the center of Amsterdam. She often finds herself on autopilot to such an extent that she can hardly recall the events of her ride upon arrival. One day she is invited to drive a Ferrari. She is proud to be able to do this; it is a childhood dream come true. Full of enthusiasm, she drives to the center of Amsterdam, but before she reaches the canals, she decides to turn around. Driving the Ferrari is much more complex than driving her regular car; she must slow down continuously. Driving demands a lot of her attention capacity, leaving her with an insufficient capacity to respond with composure to traffic situations.

A Ferrari is so fast that the driver must constantly be alerted to avoid driving too fast, in order not to create hazardous traffic situations. This is similar to the cluttering speaker. In simple (speaking) situations, it is still possible to keep one's speaking under control (on the highway, you can work with the Ferrari), but in complex situations (in the Amsterdam city center), there is insufficient attention capacity available to respond adequately; the combination of speaking and monitoring becomes too much to handle.

When working to improve speech, the client, in response to the therapist's feedback on cluttered speech, will repeat the speech models as advised by the therapist. Later, the client can recognize, detect, and correct their cluttered speech themselves, so that they will sound intelligible or fluent. In therapy, the speech therapist works toward making the feedback loop more automatic for the client. The goal of therapy for the client is to enable them to adequately plan and program their speech and language prior to execution. If a speaker has enough time for sentence formulation, the second level of monitoring can also take place in time to mitigate or eliminate mistakes in the formulation phase. As a result, audible (overt) repairs will be needed less often, and the number of word and sentence repetitions and revisions will decrease. A prerequisite for internal self-correction is to provide the speaker with sufficient time to make a correction. By slowing down the speech rate using longer pauses between speakers and sentences, the client can better plan and self-correct their speech.

Short feedback loop

"Selfcressie . . . sorry, self-correction" exemplifies a short feedback loop. This constitutes open monitoring.

Internal repair

Before articulating a multisyllabic word, the speaker attempts to slow down the rate for clearer speech intelligibility. For example: "I walk in the . . . li-bra-ry looking for a book."

Habituation

The subcomponent "habituation" needs constant attention during the treatment process. While practicing rate reduction, PWC will not feel comfortable, especially at the beginning of therapy. They will feel that their speaking is no longer "natural." This adverse reaction from the speaker will overshadow the positive effect of improved fluency and speech intelligibility.

In a group therapy session, one of the participants with cluttering uses his focused speech and is fully intelligible. Another participant remarks: "If you spoke like this all the time, your communication would improve enormously!" The first participant replies, "That may be true, but to me, it sounds so slow — I feel like a turtle. I'm not going to do that all day!"

Adopting a new speech pattern may provoke negative thoughts (for example, "It sounds strange," "People will find me boring," or "They'll think I speak too slowly,") and negative feelings, such as shame or impatience due to perceived unnatural speech.

A speech therapist should always be aware of the thoughts and negative self-evaluation of their client. The speech therapist can play segments of the client's speech using audio and video recordings, thereby showing the client that the new speech pattern is much easier to listen to. Habituation – and ultimately automation – to the "new" speech pattern is considered an essential goal of the treatment. It is very important for a speech therapist to positively encourage a client's feeling of satisfaction. Encouragement like "You have to get used to it" can often be expressed at the beginning of therapy. Later, the speech therapist may ask questions such as "Did you notice how adequately they responded to you?" or, somewhat provocatively, "And did they ask you, what are you saying?" With such casual encouragement, the resistance of the client can be reduced at an early stage so that the process of habituation can continue.

When PWC speak more slowly, fewer misarticulations and word or sentence repetitions take place, resulting in a more understandable message.

Unfortunately, people are not inclined to provide positive reinforcement for intelligible speech. The confidential advisers of the PWC play an important role. They must give positive feedback on the speech strengths where possible.

As observed, PWC often exhibit low communicative self-esteem. They can say, for example, "No one wants to hear what I have to say." In therapy, such comments should be replaced by positive encouragement, such as, "You already speak more intelligibly and fluently in many situations."

6.4.2 *The emotional component*

The affective and cognitive aspects of cluttering have not yet been extensively covered in international literature. Various authors (Bennett, 2006; Dalton & Hardcastle, 1993; Daly, 1986; Daly & Burnett, 1999; Winkelman, 1990, 1993) have emphasized that PWC can respond to their failure to speak clearly and be understood by experiencing fear, frustration (Dalton & Hardcastle, 1993), negative thoughts (Daly, 1986, 1993), nervousness, sadness, and low self-esteem (Reichel, 2010). Green (1999) suggests that speech therapists should provide positive psychosocial conditions to improve their clients' fluency and self-control skills. Langevin and Boberg (1996) suggested that their treatment should include cognitive behavioral therapy to change attitudes, perceptions, and self-confidence of PWC.

In general, the speaker and listener do not consider cluttering to be a "speech disorder" or a sign of loss of control. After all, typical disfluencies and impaired speech intelligibility generally do not interrupt communication. The lack of awareness of the symptoms as they occur prevents PWC from acknowledging problems while speaking. PWC can develop situational anxiety due to an accumulation of negative speaking experiences in a particular context (for example, constantly being interrupted while speaking at a meeting). PWC usually do not exhibit fear of specific sounds or fear of getting stuck, although a subgroup of PWC is known to fear multisyllabic words. Because PWC do not directly associate their speech with unwanted social reactions, fear of speaking will not develop quickly and will not be severe. However, sometimes, adverse reactions from listeners can give PWC communicative anxiety (experiencing fear before or during communication). The fear arises because PWC feel ignored in communicative situations and because they are frequently perceived as "noisy" or selfish. Such negative attitudes result in communication fears that can lead to avoidance and other adaptive behaviors.

Daly (1986, 1993) proposed a combination of cognitive training, counseling, attitude change, relaxation, affirmation training, and positive self-talk in working with PWC. Reichel (2010) has modified Bar-On's (2000) ten competencies related to emotional intelligence (EI) for use by speech therapists working with PWC. In her therapy approach, people with symptoms of cluttering are introduced to the following five competencies:

1. emotional self-awareness
2. impulse control
3. reality test
4. empathy
5. maintaining interpersonal relationships

The development of such skills is essential to improve awareness of emotions and communication behavior, to facilitate the ability to control emotions, achieve self-control, process emotions cognitively, assess situations realistically, and consider the feelings of listeners.

People with mild cluttering symptoms do not typically develop communicative anxiety. They predominantly exhibit the verbal-motor component. As the speech of PWC becomes more understandable, they have less communication anxiety. In moderate and severe cases of cluttering, it is especially important to work on the verbal-motor component first. You then use the cognitive component should then be used in order to interpret and reinforce the success factors. Improvements in speaking skills, as seen in PWC, enhance their awareness of their improved communication skills and increase their motivation to work further on their speech.

6.4.3   *The verbal-motor component*

Since the emotional and cognitive components of cluttering are often less severely affected than the verbal-motor component, the treatment should prioritize the verbal-motor component. In most cases, it is possible to address the high articulatory rate by slowing the speech rate with AVF (see Chapter 7, Section 7.4). Such work on speech rate reduction should be carried out in a carefully structured manner, incorporating auditory and visual feedback training.

In addition to reducing the speech rate, the speech therapist must also consider the degree of motor and linguistic demands associated with the speaking task to facilitate better coherence or synergy of speech and language output (Myers, 2011). The speech therapist must pay close attention to the levels of language complexity.

PWC are able to perform all verbal-motor movements adequately, but not when the speech rate is too fast (Van Zaalen & Winkelman, 2014).

PWC need to improve not only in the execution of oral-motor movements, such as jaw movements, but also in planning such movements. Therefore, it is essential to address verbal-motor skills at the word level. In syntactic cluttering, priority is given to the placement and duration of pauses between words and sentences. In phonological cluttering, priority is placed on accurate sequencing of syllables, especially in multisyllabic words during a fast-speaking rate. The next step is to practice such skills at the sentence level.

6.4.4 *The communicative component*

Weiss (1964) described several stigmatizing characteristics of PWC, including a lack of interest in communication, a negative attitude to life, and perceived laziness. However, it is well known that the communicative context is essential for communication between individual speakers and their interlocutors. Especially with cluttering, a period of frequent and direct feedback from the environment (partner, colleague) can contribute to an increase in speech awareness. Communicative competence is an individual skill expressed in the appropriateness of the behavior to achieve the set goal in communication and in the manner in which any miscommunications and conflicts are handled (Van Zaalen et al., 2020). This includes the following aspects:

- The client uses effective means of communication, techniques, and technology to facilitate conversations.
- The client may organize and share information with others in a manner that is respectful and appropriate and transmits it to others in a clear manner and with trust, conviction, and respect, and monitors that this information is understandable.
- The client has active listening skills and stimulates the ideas and opinions of others.
- The client can give feedback and receive it respectfully and integrate received feedback into their speech.
- The client recognizes how diversity in experience, expertise, culture, and hierarchy within a relationship can contribute to effective communication, conflict management, and a positive relationship.

To explain these aspects, therapists should familiarize themselves with Interprofessional Communication in Care and Welfare (Van Zaalen et al., 2020). Partner-oriented communication (adapting the message to the listener) is a skill that can be further developed in PWC.

Dysfunctional communication, characterized by poor listening, abnormal turn-taking behavior, and verbosity, can occur in PWC, especially during moments of heightened emotional arousal. Above all, the level of relationship is mainly determined by mental linguistic, and nonverbal behavior, such as mimicry, loudness, pausing, stress, and gestures. PWC can send unintended

and unwanted messages. Unfortunately, this has led in the past to misinter-
pretations of the personalities of PWC as described by Weiss (1964), which
have been repeated many times in subsequent publications in the twentieth
century.

6.4.5   *Therapeutic considerations*

Planning a cluttering intervention depends on the results of the comprehensive evaluation and assessment of the diagnostic exercises. Treatment of PWC
requires a clear structure. The client should practice daily, starting on the first
day of therapy, according to the SMART criteria. It is also critical that the
amount of exercise per day is tailored to each client's symptoms, skill level,
and needs. Treatment plans for syntactic (see Chapter 7, Section 7.5) and
phonological cluttering always start with identification exercises (see Chapter 7, Section 7.6; and for subtyping, see Chapter 1, Section 1.4.10). It is
unnecessary to do all the identification exercises with each client. After the
identification stage, exercises for adjusting the speech rate will be discussed
(see Chapter 7, Sections 7.5.4 and 7.6.4). Suggestions on how to work on
language formulation and story building (Chapter 7, Section 7.5.5) and on
prosody, speech rhythm, and melody (Chapter 7, Section 7.6.5) will also be
provided.

It is crucial to praise and validate PWC every time a goal is achieved. The
sense of success and being on the journey together will bring PWC hope,
pride, and courage to try to overcome their remaining symptoms of cluttering. Special attention must be paid to increasing speech awareness and improving pragmatic skills such as taking turns, maintaining topics, and telling
stories. The choice of therapy method is determined by the clients' knowledge obtained during the diagnostic exercises and their personal interests.
Syllable tapping is particularly recommended at the word level, especially
with multisyllable words. AVF training (see Chapter 7, Section 7.4) is advised for improving comprehensibility and intelligibility at the sentence level.
Mindfulness exercises (see Chapter 7, Section 7.9) will positively affect inner
peace and, thus, the duration of focused attention.

For example, the speech therapist chooses the AVF training with young
people and adults who like to work with computers. The convenience of
syllable tapping is that it can be used at any time while the client is speaking. Once syllable awareness is achieved at different levels of linguistic complexity, the speech therapist can use AVF training to work on rate, rhythm,
pauses, and prosody. When providing therapy to people not interested in
working with AVF, there are alternative, more traditional, but less sustainable methods of achieving their goals.

Another important consideration when selecting which approach to take
for lowering the speech rate is whether the client's cluttering is accompanied
by stuttering. People with cluttering-stuttering would probably get the maximum benefit from AVF training because syllable tapping carries the risk that

individuals who stutter will exhibit secondary behaviors when performed incorrectly. In individuals with high levels of physical restlessness, mindfulness exercises can be helpful in finding the right state of mind to perform identification and monitoring exercises.

6.5 Practice hierarchy

To determine the order of the speaking situations in which the exercises are performed, a client should complete the Speech Situation Checklist by Brutten (1979), which is modified to cluttering (see Appendix I). When this is done, both the client and the speech therapist can better understand the client's ability to communicate in different conversational situations. Without a doubt, the exercises will be done first in those speaking situations that are known to pose fewer problems. By doing so, a client can be successful early in the short term, and that success (and each subsequent success) will strengthen their internal motivation to change. The speech therapist will also determine which level of language complexity needs to be addressed first.

Finally, a list of perceived feelings and emotions should be discussed (see Appendix I). This completed list makes clients aware of their negative thoughts and feelings regarding their speech and general communication.

Table 6.1 Therapeutic prioritization based on the severity of cluttering symptoms in various speaking situations.

The score for cluttering experience in a specific speaking situation	The score for emotional or cognitive experiences	Implication to therapy
Speaking situations in which no or hardly any cluttering symptoms are present (score of 0 or 1)		No therapy needed
Speaking situations in which some cluttering symptoms are reported (score of 2 and 3)	Mild emotional or cognitive response (0 and 1)	Step 1
Speaking situations in which mild to moderate cluttering symptoms are reported (score of 3 or 4)	Moderate to severe emotional or cognitive response (> 2)	Step 2
Speaking situations in which moderate to severe cluttering symptoms are reported (score of 4 and 5)	Mild emotional or cognitive responses (0 and 1)	Step 3
Speaking situations in which severe cluttering symptoms are reported (score of 5 and 6)	Moderate to severe emotional or cognitive responses (score > 2)	Step 4

Note, it will be determined at which levels of language complexity each task should be practiced. For example, if certain speaking situations do not take place in the life of the client, the therapy will consist of fewer steps.

If the therapy is ongoing, the Cluttering Assessment Battery and the Speech Situation Checklist can be re-administered to measure the efficacy of the intervention.

6.6   Intensity of treatment

Planning an intensive intervention program is recommended for cluttering therapy to be successful. Self-control skills take time to develop and are acquired with intense exercise (Bennett Lanouette, 2011). Motor learning is complex and has many aspects. This section will discuss the main aspects of motor learning.

1   *Intensive practice*

No studies on the treatment efficacy of cluttering were conducted until Van Zaalen and Reichel (2014) presented a study evaluating the efficacy of the intensive intervention on cluttering.

One can also learn from additional studies on the efficacy of speech motor learning, such as a study on Parkinson's disease. A meta-analysis by Kaipa et al. (2016) on individuals with Parkinson's suggests that repeated practice facilitates speech-motor learning regardless of the type of exercise.

2   *The importance of an external focus of attention*

What should clients with cluttering focus their attention on while performing and learning motor speaking tasks? Should they pay attention to the execution of their movements or their effects on the environment? Or does this depend on the task and the individual?

Audio-visual feedback is a form of "knowledge of performance" (KP). Another type of feedback is called "knowledge of results" (KR). It is preferably given at three levels (for example, "correct," "almost right," and "incorrect") within two to three seconds after the production of the client (Steinberg, Lowe & Buchwald, 2017). KR feedback of "almost good" is given if only one phoneme is produced incorrectly or if, although all phonemes are accurate, speech production is not fluent.

3   *The importance of explicit knowledge building*

What kind of instructions should speech therapists give to PWC? For example, should they give explicit instructions on how movements should be performed? Or are more implicit forms of learning and instruction preferable?

In order to assist clients to make adjustments in their speech and achieve their SMART goals, clinicians must provide detailed directions and objective feedback. It is not prudent to rely solely on the expertise of the speech therapist. As noted above, a clinician's interpretation of the rate is influenced by their client's dialect, energy level, age, and familiarity with the content of the task. It is essential for the client to know objectively what needs to be changed about their speech. Measuring changes in speech production provides clients with the opportunity for self-management. Less intensive approaches do not provide the opportunity to facilitate new speaking patterns. Practicing new skills in a speech therapy clinic is not enough. The new speaking patterns must be integrated into daily communication. The actual exercises should occur in all settings where a person speaks — at home, at work, on the road, during sports training, and so on. Speech therapists should candidly inform their clients who have cluttering that maintaining control of their speech quality in every situation can be highly challenging. However, they should not let this discourage them. Even though most people with cluttering cannot monitor their speech in every situation, speaking with clarity is always important. This is true even if it is only achievable in a few speaking situations (Miyamoto, 2011).

4   *The importance of contextual interference*

How vital is variation during practice for learning motor skills? Is it best to continuously repeat movement techniques to become well automated?

Contextual interference (CI) is preferred: practicing motor movements in a random order, may interfere with each other. In other words, phonetic training has little value, while practicing speech in complex word sequences can be of great value. Video training with contextual interference in sports improves more than inconsistent training, both in recognizing and correcting errors. Practicing syllables "dry" several times in speech therapy might not necessarily lead to their transferring into spontaneous speech. However, words practiced with stressing of syllables can be correctly implemented. This method also influences words that have not yet been practiced, especially when the practice is supplemented with AVF. Practical experience suggests that this is indeed true for the pronunciation of multisyllabic words, but further research is needed to confirm this assumption.

5   *The importance of random variations in execution*

Should PWC always try to get as close as possible to the correct externally prescribed technique so this "'ideal of movement" becomes increasingly "established"? Or would it be beneficial to vary the execution method considerably for the brain to learn from differences and discover the optimal speaking technique itself? In many speech treatments, speech therapists use isolated exercises. The literature on motor learning clearly shows that isolated exercises, while facilitating the acquisition of target behavior, do not lead to generalization. Research shows that random exercise facilitates stabilization, while isolated exercises do not (Knock et al., 2000). For cluttering therapy, this means that working on isolated exercises does not provide sufficient stabilization. We advocate practicing in a communicative context because these random variations in the execution are necessary for the stabilization of automatically produced speech. This is done, for example, by including and analyzing conversations in daily communications. (See also Chapter 7, Section 7.4.)

6   *Fast technique correction with old way – new way*

After many years of training, clients have developed an abnormal movement technique that limits their performance. How can this incorrect technique (old way) be replaced by a new, better technique (new way) without the old technique occasionally reemerging? Clients with phonological cluttering will have difficulty producing words that they regularly use – for example, their own names or professional jargon – in the right way. After all, the old way is stored in their lexical memory. Awareness of the mistake is made, and repeated identification of this error in the communicative context requires extra attention. This also involves a more extended period of monitoring. Clients with syntactic cluttering often begin speaking before the formulation of the sentence is sufficiently prepared. After a few words, time is gained by utilizing typical disfluencies. This tendency must be nipped in the bud. Once this happens, interrupt the client, and ask them to take enough time for the formulation of their idea and only then start speaking.

7   *Practice in combination with sleeping makes perfect*

A good night's sleep is crucial for performance, but what is the relationship between motor learning and sleep? Can sleep promote motor learning and thus help improve the performance of clients with cluttering? If so, how?

It is too early to make firm statements about the relationship between sleep and motor learning. However, intensive practice is exhausting, and a short or power nap could actively contribute to improved speech control for clients.

8   *The importance of observing and imitating*

Why is imitating modeled behavior a basic form of learning in humans and animals? What are the cognitive and neural bases for that? How can PWC and speech therapists benefit from scientific insights in this area?

A common remark by some PWC is, "But I still had enough breath; I didn't need to stop." The client who says or does this can learn by observing others; for example, PRAAT demonstrates the pauses that a speech therapist makes. However, taking note of pauses can also be helpful within home or school situations. When clients make little to no pauses, it is important for them to continue observing the pauses of others until they conclude that "others actually take pauses very often" (identification).

9 The importance of self-management

Speech therapists can guide the motor learning processes, but PWC can also self-direct these processes. Unfortunately, research results in this area are still scarce. The initial study on AVF training for cluttering (Van Zaalen & Reichel, 2014) has shown that self-management by PWC is positively received and contributes to consistent intervention effectiveness. Self-management means that the PWC feel that they are in control of their speech. Developing self-direction is essential to be successful in life, especially for a person dealing with a chronic condition such as cluttering.

10 Individual differences and learning styles

People speak differently, but do they also learn differently? If so, what are these differences, and what empirical evidence supports them? Should speech therapists make their training methods depend on the individual clients with cluttering? It is known from the behavioral sciences and motor-learning theories that the period for maintaining the newly acquired behavior is expected to vary from 10 to 12 weeks. The time required for changes in speaking behavior is related to the functioning of the cerebellum, and more specifically to neuroplasticity. Just as the cerebellum maintains balance, integration, and stability in the somatic-motor sphere, it can also help balance, integrate, and stabilize other brain functions (Rapoport et al., 2000).

Neuroplasticity is the brain's natural ability to reorganize itself by forming new neural pathways and connections throughout life. Neuroplasticity allows the brain's nerve cells (neurons) to adjust their functioning in response to new situations or changes in their environment to compensate for existing problems. Cortical representation is strengthened and enlarged when a stimulus is cognitively associated with amplification. In some cases, cortical representations can double or triple in one or two days when a new sensorimotor behavior is first acquired, and changes are primarily completed within a few weeks at most (Blake et al., 2006). Exercises should therefore be performed often (five times a day) and for a short time (10 to 12 weeks). After all, no learned habit or skill of people is as frequent as speech. Usually, the old habits are maintained during the day. This means that the time in which the new habit is practiced is relatively limited. Only intensive practice can compete with this.

An intensive training schedule is necessary for PWC to compensate for their limited self-awareness and weak symptom awareness. Because monitoring in PWC is weak, they need assistance in establishing voice control. It is also more difficult for them to acquire an internal locus of control, in order to get the feeling that they are able to improve their communication.

6.7   SMART criteria

A treatment goal is the desired outcome of a treatment plan, which is considered an intermediate operational step to achieve the ultimate objective of a treatment program. A session goal or practice goal is one of the steps to achieve the treatment goal. Whether assignments and exercises yield results depends on whether they are executed within a clear framework. The exercises must therefore meet specific criteria. In the case of cluttering, each practice assignment must be described to the client as clearly as possible. SMART criteria are an effective means to achieve this goal. The acronym SMART stands for:

- specific
- measurable
- acceptable
- realistic
- time-bound

For everyday use, these SMART criteria are intended as a guide. They sometimes overlap. If exercises do not meet the SMART criteria, there is a good chance that the clients will not be trained efficiently. This means that a positive outcome of the exercise becomes highly unlikely; consequently, speech therapy might then be perceived as a burden, leading to a decrease in motivation. Next, the SMART criteria specific to cluttering are discussed. The SMART criteria are explained below as they apply to both homework assignments and the completion of self-observation schedules (see Section 6.9).

6.7.1   *Specific*

"Specific" refers to the ability of clients to evaluate the (sub)purpose of each exercise precisely. Speech therapists should avoid making their objectives open to multiple interpretations. It is helpful to describe therapy objectives to clients and to ask them to indicate in their own words what will be worked on. If objectives align with clients' perspectives on treatment, the objectives should be pursued. For example, the self-identification of a symptom by a client is an important condition to achieve the goal of the identification phase of treatment. Identification exercises should be performed at home without the help of the speech therapist. If clients are unable to identify their symptoms, this exercise is useless.

For instance, if the syllable typing exercise needs clarification for successful home assignments, the cluttering is likely to persist. The purpose of an assignment must be clear, unambiguous, and positively formulated. In each exercise, the following questions need to be answered: "What?", "Why?", "When?", "How?", "How long?" and "How often?" Generally, the exercises should be practiced often and for a short time.

The following example clarifies how giving a specific and measurable assignment can influence clients with cluttering.

A specific assignment

Lloyd, a 12-year-old boy, is instructed by his speech therapist to record his speech daily to determine his articulatory rate using Talk. Lloyd is asked to calculate fragments of 10 to 20 consecutive flowing syllables without pauses. The goal is to achieve an average articulatory rate of 5.5 to 6.5 SPS, as calculated over five attempts. In addition, the variation between the highest and lowest scores should not exceed 2 SPS. Lloyd enters the therapy room for the next session smiling and immediately begins discussing his home assignment. He has found that he achieved his goal at least once a day, and sometimes even twice a day. He thinks about doing it again and strives to reach his goal twice a day within a week.

6.7.2 Measurable

The results of the performance of exercises must be measurable. This means that the speech therapist and the client can objectively determine whether the goal of the exercise has been achieved. For each exercise, make sure it is clear how the result can be interpreted in percentages or absolute numbers. For example: "In 16 out of 20 sentences, pauses are made in linguistically correct places." This implementation can be achieved in many ways. Alternatively: "the average articulatory rate fell in the range of 5.6 to 6.6 SPS." PRAAT software provides the possibility to take objective measurements. Detailed instructions for PRAAT Software can be found in Chapter 7, Sections 7.4–7.6. The use of a self-observation schedule is one method to make activities visible and measurable for both the client and the speech therapist. Providing ranges of desired scores allows the objective measurements to reflect the development within a specific practice goal (for example, see Table 6.2).

Table 6.2 Speaking observation assignment completion diagram (example)

While simulating a broadcast, the client's articulation rate within the target area ranges from 4.8–5.9 SPS. When reaching four out of five correct productions (80%) over five consecutive days, practice can be performed within a more complex context (either a challenging speaking situation or a higher level of language complexity).

Name: Diego

Date	Measurement 1	Measurement 2	Measurement 3	Measurement 4	Measurement 5	Goal achieved	Remarks
Sept 23	6.23	7.3	5.8	7.9	6.8	1/5	Sometimes misunderstood
Sept 24	6.43	6.2	6.1	6.5	6.4	0/5	Few repeats necessary
Sept 25	5.47	6.4	5.8	5.9	5.2	4/5	Nice talk

Note: White area: > 6.8 SPS; light gray area: 5.8–6.7; dark grey area (target area): 4.8–5.9 SPS. Areas have been drawn up for this specific client based on multiple measurements within the speaking situation.

Again, the purpose of the assignment must be clearly and positively formulated. Here are some examples of acceptable criteria:

- Number of errors in 100 words per minute.
- Articulatory rate in syllables per second.
- Pause duration of 0.5–1.0 seconds between sentences.

6.7.3 *Acceptable*

Is the intended result acceptable to the effort that the client thinks they are expected to make? Does everyone involved agree on this? As the client learns to speak differently, they generally find that a lot of attention capacity is needed to change their speaking. The effort exerted by the client must outweigh the added value gained from communication within the environment. It is, therefore, essential to assess the following two things in each exercise: The adjustments in speaking and their effect on communication. The effect on communication is determined based on comprehensibility and intelligibility. Since we cannot always ask the listener whether a message has been understood, the effect is measured based on appropriate responses, the lack of questions for repetition, the lack of "What do you say?", and so forth. If an exercise is unacceptable to the client, they will not do it at home. The sub-goal should be emphasized in each exercise (See the example below).

An acceptable target for syllable tapping

While on the phone, ensure that every syllable is audible in the first 30 seconds. After 30 seconds, the client should continue to speak without this additional focus. When playing back the phone call recording, the client should listen to determine how long they are able to produce sentences in which all syllables are audible.

An assignment should focus on the perception of the moment. Block (2004) advocates person-centered therapy, even if the speech therapist must work against an evidence-based approach. Block recommends that the speech therapist should discuss the new speech pattern to habituate the client to their newly acquired, natural-sounding speech, even if it does not feel natural.

Clients who do not practice often enough should be asked what they plan to change in the coming week to encourage more frequent practice. If the client does not like the treatment offered by their speech therapist, it is irrelevant to what the supporting evidence indicates; people will not choose to use them (Block, 2004). If an exercise is not yet feasible but is needed to continue the process, the resistance of the client must be addressed, for example, with cognitive restructuring. The exercise can be made more realistic by emphasizing the purpose of the session.

"Exercise motivation" and "therapy loyalty" are strongly related to the criteria determining which goals are "acceptable." To illustrate, many people want to learn how to draw, but only a few are willing to sit down and try it for a long time.

6.7.4   Realistic

If the speech therapist in the earlier example (See Table 6.2) selects a range of 4.5–5.0 SPS as the target area, this means that the client did not meet the target in any of the cases. Despite the discipline showed by practicing fifteen times, the goal was never met. That is not motivating. The thought, "I'll never succeed," can come to mind to this client. Although it may ultimately be the case that the client is best understood or understandable within the range of 4.5–5.0 SPS, that is not a realistic goal at this point in treating the client. The range should always be based on values already established to reduce the likelihood that the client will drop out.

The exercises designed to facilitate the selected behavior should also fit easily into the client's daily routine. For example, clients who work in an office can easily have short conversations with several colleagues throughout the day and incorporate exercises into those interactions. While asking a student to call someone five times a day may be unrealistic, it can be more feasible to ask a student to initiate a fluent sentence five times during an online computer game. Thus, the speech therapist needs to be realistic in understanding the potential skills of the client, taking the following considerations into account:

- making few or no demands does not lead to improvement;
- demands that are too high can lead to a lack of success in therapy;
- taking too big a step can lead to disappointment. On the other hand, a lack of success in therapy does not always cause disappointment but can also arise from the client's having expectations that are unreasonably high or the client's staying at the same level for too long;
- intensive practice is only possible if it happens within everyday events;
- practicing only at the table is not communication.

Cognitive psychology defines how people explain their behavior from the so-called locus of control perspective. When people are deeply convinced that the condition of cluttering inevitably controls them, this is referred to as having an "external locus of control." When people have such beliefs, intervention objectives have little chance of success. On the other hand, people with a high "internal locus of control" are convinced that they can change their behavior themselves. This generally leads to a greater chance of a successful intervention outcome.

> An assignment must be difficult enough to be a challenge and easy enough to enable the client to achieve the goal (Zaalen & Winkelman, 2014).

Internal attribution is the way that some people interpret a person's behavior and emphasize certain personality traits. If someone stumbles, for example, others may conclude that it is because the person who stumbled is clumsy. When individuals take responsibility for their actions and firmly believe they are responsible for their own actions, they have an internal locus of control. For example, PWC with an internal locus of control are able to say, "If I practice enough, I can adjust my speech."

6.7.5 Time-bound

The speech therapist should clarify to the client how long the therapy program will last. Long-term goals can be planned over a more extended period. Short-term goals can be planned for a shorter and specific period, such as within a week. A clear schedule should be established regarding the duration and frequency of therapy sessions. If clients follow this schedule, the therapy is likely to be more sustainable, and its outcome can be more easily evaluated. As discussed earlier, cluttering therapy should be intensive. This principle also applies to the planning of assignments. In most cases, the exercises must be performed frequently but scheduled for short periods.

Examples of time schedules for assignments timetables

- Five minutes every day, for a week
- Every fifteen minutes for one minute
- Only in certain communicative situations; for example, during telephone conversations
- Only with a certain person
- In the first two minutes of each conversation
- When shopping

6.8   Practice assignments

The speech therapist should make the practice assignments as engaging as possible and should also discuss how to best perform the exercises, who can be the best conversational partner, how to make audio or video recordings, and how to conduct an ideal evaluation. The therapist can ask questions like "What is the purpose of this exercise?", Did you achieve your goal?", and "Are you satisfied with the number of times you recorded and analyzed your sentences?" Such questions can provide deep insights into the value of exercise. To encourage clients to complete their exercises, they can set up reminders as a tool. For example, set the alarm clock on a mobile phone every hour, several times a day, or in certain situations (for example, at a party or a business meeting) as a reminder. Use the vibration function so that others are not disturbed by the reminder. Clients are reminded of the practice assignment and the points they must focus on each time they receive such a memo. Displaying the exercise results, along with the date, subject, and level of language complexity, provides clients with insights into their progress.

6.9   Self-observation schemes

Self-observation schemes help clients become aware of the differences between their old and new behavior. Such schemes can be used during the pre-assessment, as well as during therapy. In the assessment phase, the clients must keep schedules daily and, on some days, even every hour. In the therapy phase, this can be done less often. During the therapy phase, the speech therapist may also ask the client to pay attention to only one aspect of speech. In the self-observation diagrams, the following observation objectives can be instructive:

- How many times per minute is a repetition audible?
- How many times per minute do the clients say "uhm"?
- To which pronunciation of words does the listener look puzzled?
- How often does the listener respond appropriately to the story being told?

As suggested above, the frequency of completing the schedules can vary from once a day to – in the cases where necessary – every hour. In the therapeutic phase, the designated goals can be set less often, or specific exercises can sometimes be limited to specific goals. However, the sessions should not be scheduled too frequently, because doing so could cause the therapy to be perceived as too much of a chore.

6.10   Summary

This chapter discusses the treatment of cluttering, and describes, among other things, changes in social communication, problems with monitoring, priorities in treatment, exercise hierarchy, and the intensity of treatment. This chapter also describes what progress can be expected in the short and long term and how these effects can be stabilized. The chapter continues with an appreciation of an intensive training schedule and discusses the importance of integrating a new speech pattern into daily communication so that PWC can compensate for their limited symptom awareness and monitoring skills. Finally, the chapter ends with a discussion of SMART goals within cluttering therapy.

7 Therapy methods and exercises

7.1 Identification

A wide range of treatment approaches can be used in cluttering therapy. The decision about which approach to use depends on the symptoms and the ability to address the needs of the client. The means of intervention must be compatible with the experiences and abilities of clients. Cluttering therapy always starts with the identification stage, which means becoming aware of the symptoms as they occur. By making clients aware of their symptoms, speech therapists can discuss the effects of poor intelligibility or disfluencies on their clients and their listeners. Such a discussion about speaking behavior can change the clients' perception of themselves as communication partners. This is the right time to encourage clients to adapt their communication patterns in order to reduce their symptoms related to cluttering. Understanding how fast their speech rate is will encourage clients to use strategies for lowering that rate. After clients become aware of their speech and language symptoms, they can be trained to take appropriate pauses.

Focused attention is considered a controlled process. Controlled processes are intentional, controllable, persistent, and consciously implemented (Bargh, 1994; Johnson & Hasher, 1987; Kahneman & Treisman, 1984; Logan & Cowan, 1984). Such a consciously controlled process uses a segment of attention that would otherwise be used for other processes, such as language formulation. Too much focus on speech production, however, can have a negative effect on language formulation in linguistically complex conditions. At the same time, too much focus on language formulation can have a negative effect on speech production. As described in Chapter 6, Section 6.5, the practice should be organized within a hierarchy. The practice hierarchy should consider the speaking situation, the emotional response, and the level of language complexity. Never ask clients with cluttering to apply strategies at a level where the goal is not achievable. The levels of language complexity are discussed in Section 7.2. Identification exercises are elaborated on in Sections 7.5.1 to 7.5.3, 7.6.1, and 7.6.2. Before this, section 7.1 examines the necessity of identification of symptoms of cluttering. The

DOI: 10.4324/9781003460558-10

last sections of this chapter describe the therapy for syntactic cluttering (Section 7.5), phonological cluttering (Section 7.6), and cluttering-stuttering (Section 7.7). In addition to the AVF training described in Section 7.4, syllable tapping (Section 7.8) and the value of mindfulness (section 7.9) in cluttering therapy are examined.

7.1.1 The role of the environment in the identification

People in the immediate environment of PWC tend to make many comments about the speech behavior of people with this condition, without any positive effect, and to the contrary, frequently cause distress. Often, PWC are asked, 'Speak clearly!' 'Slower!' or similar comments, all intended to change the speech of PWC. PWC need to understand these well-intentioned comments because, in their own perception, they speak calmly, comprehensibly, and intelligibly. Over time, these comments can take on a negative connotation. Speech therapists must gain and maintain the trust of their clients so that the speech therapists' feedback is believed and accepted by their clients and will subsequently lead to a positive change in the behavior of their clients. This is achieved on the one hand by giving objective feedback to the clients and, on the other hand, by rewarding desired behaviors and identifying undesirable behaviors in a ratio of 5:1.

It is best to start therapy by educating PWC and people close to them about cluttering. It is advisable to include people from the immediate environment of the PWC, such as parents, partners, teachers, or a colleague, as soon as possible. Family members and other people close to the PWC can alert their child, partner, or colleague about the cluttering symptoms and in this way can help develop symptom awareness. An additional benefit is that people close to the PWC no longer feel that nothing can be done about the hasty or unintelligible speech of the PWC. The best way to help PWC is for the people close to them to ask more often:

"I heard [. . .]. Is that what you wanted to say?"

or:

"I believe you want to say [. . .]. Did I understand that correctly?"

or variations of these two examples.

By asking these or similar questions, listeners no longer resign themselves to misinterpreting the unclear message, and concurrently, the PWC learn to speak with greater awareness.

7.1.2   External feedback

In conversations with PWC and the people around them, clear arrangements should be made about how the comments are to be given. Confidants can, for example, create a pre-arranged audible or visual sign that can be used up to a certain number of times during the day.

> **Visual support feedback**
>
> Stick magnets on the refrigerator. Each time feedback is given, a magnet is removed from the refrigerator and set aside. If no more magnets are on the refrigerator, no more verbal feedback will be given that day.

A second arrangement can be made about giving feedback when other people are within hearing range. Preferably, the feedback on the quality of the speech is not directly observable or audible to the other listeners.

Finally, it is important to ensure that PWC believe that feedback from those around them is genuinely honest, caring, and constructive. Only with that trust, when feedback is given, will PWC respond without anger or frustration and instead modify their behavior. The feedback from loved ones contributes to a more effective feedback loop. PWC must be corrected and often complimented, especially when they correct their speech on their own, i.e., without suggestions from people close to them. In this way, the internalization of monitoring will develop faster.

During the process of internalizing monitoring, external sound sources can be confusing. For instance, with an unfavorable signal-to-noise ratio, speech can become less intelligible if someone is standing near a music source or an open window. This is especially true when speaking on a mobile phone or during a video call. PWC can be made aware of these challenges and should learn to speak louder or more clearly in such situations. These suggestions can positively affect speech clarity in cases where the signal-to-noise ratio is unfavorable for intelligibility.

7.1.3   Monitoring by identification

PWC need to learn to listen critically to their speech and thereby recognize moments of improved comprehensibility and intelligibility. The identification phase of the treatment can begin by having the client listen to a recording of their speech, which is preferably made without the client being aware of it being recorded. The speech therapist may ask the client to call friends and record those phone calls. In general, clients are no longer focused on the recording after 30 to 40 seconds; they continue to chat with their friends naturally. Such conversations often include cluttering symptoms. Listening to and analyzing their own recordings becomes more challenging when it continues for a period of several minutes or the recording was made a few days earlier.

When listening to these longer or older recordings, clients may forget the original context, which makes the errors in their speech more apparent to the clients as listeners. Having the clients listen to their own recordings is a very effective and efficient homework assignment. Ensuring that the practice assignment meets the SMART criteria (see Chapter 6, Section 6.7) is important. For example, clients should be given very specific instructions, such as:

• how many recordings they have to make;
• how many times a day;
• how long the recordings should take;
• on which criteria these recordings will be evaluated.

In the next session, the perception of the client can be compared with that of the speech therapist. After the client listens to the recording, the identification training can be scheduled with different subgoals.

7.1.4 Development of the feedback loop

Throughout treatment, identifying cluttering symptoms should be an important point of attention. Clients need to be taught how to recognize their symptoms and understand (from an internal locus of control) what they can change about their speech on their own. Developing the so-called internal feedback loop is often very slow. This loop consists of the elements of self-observation, self-judgment, and self-correction. (See Levelt's language production model in Chapter 1, Section 1.6.) When training the feedback loop as a self-monitoring technique, two goals must be met:

• Subgoal 1: Improve self-awareness at the sensory level. Rhythm, speed, timing, and kinesthetic awareness play a role.
• Subgoal 2: Improve phonological planning skills.

Often, clients become aware of their 'abnormal' speech only after the end of communication; for example, after completing a sentence and noticing a listener's frown, or even at the end of a conversation. The AVF training (see Section 7.4) can help PWC by providing feedback immediately after the moment of motor execution and speech production or even in real-time (i.e., during speech production). The AVF training allows clients to analyze their own speech within the normal (listener) range. This is essential because the most challenging aspect of changing speech behavior in cluttering is that the PWC perceive their rate as normal and their speech as fluent and intelligible.

> The AVF training enables PWC to respond correctly to their speech characteristics and to create a frame of reference where their speech is intelligible and fluent.

Once PWC can identify differences in their speech rate, work can start on slowing down their articulatory rate.

There are three ways to reduce the articulatory rate: AVF training (see Section 7.4), syllable tapping (see Section 7.8), and mindfulness (see Section 7.9).

7.2   Levels of language complexity

If clients can adequately identify their symptoms and pay attention to the appropriate speech characteristics, the speech therapist can work on implementing what has been learned in controlled speaking situations. PWC should be encouraged to focus intensely because good concentration improves clients' ability to monitor their speech performance during complex language formulation tasks. The speech therapist needs to choose exercises that have a higher language complexity than was previously possible. Training language production under more complex conditions might reduce the dissynchronicity between language formulation and speech production. Speech therapists will keep the different levels of language complexity in mind when planning the assessment and therapy exercises. The ultimate goal is to enable clients to control their speech at all levels of language complexity.

> **Hierarchy of different levels of language complexity**
>
> 1. Listing (7.2.1)
> 2. Reading (7.2.2)
> 3. Describing (7.2.3)
> 4. Retelling (7.2.4)
> 5. Telling a story (7.2.5)
> 6. Explaining (7.2.6)
> 7. Associative storytelling (7.2.7)
> 8. Level 1–6, focusing on abstract concepts (7.2.8)
> 9. Discussing (7.2.9)
> 10. Persuading (7.2.10)
>
> Note: In all exercises, the ultimate goal is to achieve the appropriate speaking goal for the PWC at the relevant level of language complexity.

7.2.1 Listing

When listing, the client often speaks at the word level. Words from the same semantic or phonological categories are often used, making the retrieval of appropriate motor programs easier.

Exercise A

Name as many names of girls in your class as possible.

Exercise B

Name as many countries as possible where English is spoken.

Exercise C

Name as many words as possible related to the Christmas holidays.

7.2.2 Reading

Reading involves phonological processes, speech-motor planning, and execution. After all, nothing needs to be formulated; this has already been done by the writer of the reading material. When reading unfamiliar texts, clients can focus easily on the words they produce. When rereading a text, the focus may decrease, leading to more errors. The errors are expected to occur mainly with the small words (less focus) and less with the multisyllabic words. Reading texts with higher complexity aloud will also generate more focus for clients, so these types of texts are recommended over simple texts. Which texts are considered complex for an individual client can be determined by trying different texts. The sentence length, the length of the words, and the number of consonant clusters per syllable usually determine the degree of complexity. When choosing a text, a limit of 95 percent accuracy of reading aloud is generally recommended. This is based on the suggestions for reading offered by Allington et al., 2015):

- *Focused attention.* Allington et al. support the idea that having students read texts with an accuracy of at least 95 percent can lead to greater gains in behavior, task orientation, and text comprehension compared to reading too difficult texts.
- *Vocabulary acquisition.* Independent reading is the source of the largest vocabulary acquisition. However, if a text contains many unfamiliar words, the context will need to be stronger even to facilitate word recognition and to learn the new word's meaning. A complex text will facilitate more focus in clients with cluttering.
- *Self-regulation behavior.* Readers use self-correction strategies and try to use graphic cues to decode unfamiliar words when reading material with at least 95 percent accuracy.

> When practicing reading, the goal should not be learning to read better but gaining the ability to slow down the rate of reading.

Exercise A

Ask the client to read a news item from a news app or a tear-off calendar. The advantage of using such an app is that a new reading text is always available with little effort. The client makes a recording of the reading with the mobile phone and assesses it immediately after recording the predetermined speaking goals. If the client is satisfied, the exercise stops. If the client is not satisfied, they will make a second recording.

Exercise B

Ask the client to read aloud all the texts that appear on the screen during a game. Then ask the client to make recordings of them reading with the PRAAT software, and after the game is completed, analyze the recordings with mutually agreed speech goals. These are easily found in the full recording by writing down the time it took to read each text on the screen.

Exercise C

During choral reading, the client must adjust their rate of reading to the speech therapist's rate. When the client reaches the right rate, the speech therapist reads softer and softer, until they are barely audible. If the client goes too fast again (speech becomes unintelligible or disfluent), the speech therapist reads louder again. After three minutes of reading, the recording is played back, and the speech is analyzed in segments where the speech therapist is barely audible or not audible at all.

7.2.3 Describing

When describing images, using photographs, paintings, or other works of art, the client will tend to speak in relatively short sentences. Additional pauses between statements may be observed. Sometimes this means that the client is searching for the right words, which will slow things down. In cases of syntactic cluttering, this can trigger additional typical disfluencies. If that happens, give the client more time to think before they start speaking.

Exercise A

The speech therapist asks the client to imagine a picture and describe it to someone who cannot see the picture. In the beginning, no restrictions should be imposed. After some time, when a client can perform this exercise fluently and intelligibly, the speech therapist gives the client some words that should not be used while describing the image. The purpose of these taboo words is to strengthen internal focus and improve the likelihood of inhibition while describing a picture.

Exercise B

When formulating language, a client should not only focus on what they say or how they express themselves, but they must also draw on their memory. When the speech therapist asks the client to examine a busy photo for a few minutes before describing what they have observed, the attention is partially shifted away from their memory.

Exercise C

Ask the client to describe the layout of their home. Ask them to do this in such detail that the speech therapist can make a drawing of it.

Describing funny images

Description exercises can be made more difficult by using 'fun photos' with bizarre details. This requires sharing more information, so the message gets across to the listener. It also challenges the listener's memory.

Exercise A

The client describes a photo, and the speech therapist chooses the right photo from several similar photos.

Exercise B

Identifying small visual changes, such as pointing out four differences in photographs presented, is more difficult than merely describing what the client sees. The speech therapist can use various computer games, such as The Puzzle Maker (2021), or create photos with minor differences. To do this, the client simply needs to remove elements from an illustration and fill in the gaps with the color of the surrounding environment.

The client is asked to describe the differences in clearly produced complete sentences. Since the game is not the goal, but only a procedure to achieve a goal, it is best for speech therapists not to give this exercise as a home assignment. If the game is given as a home assignment, there is a high likelihood that the client will play the game on their own without using it as an exercise to adjust the speech and articulatory rate to the linguistic demands needed for the exercise completion.

7.2.4 *Retelling*

When retelling a story, the client can use existing language constructs from memory. This certainly plays a role if the time between the first narration and the retelling is limited, as is the case with retelling the Wallet Story from the Cluttering Assessment Battery. Because less attention capacity is needed to formulate the sentences and because the story structure is already provided, more attention capacity remains for the client to focus on speech and language production.

Exercise A

The client is asked to share daily experiences with the speech therapist, a family member, or a partner.

Exercise B

Ask the client to read a short news story and retell it. If the client is open to this, you can also give the assignment to provide additional focus to speaking daily when telling at least one news event.

7.2.5 *Storytelling*

The narration starts with the conceptualization in Levelt's model of language production (see Figure 1.8 in Chapter 1). The client tries to convey an idea or an experience to the listener. Particular attention will be paid to the story's introduction and the storyline. It is easier for the client to tell a story about an experience that involves a certain amount of emotion. The content of the message is determined entirely by what the client chooses to share or withhold. All sentences are formulated and planned during the telling of a story. The PWC must consider the listener's prior knowledge.

Exercise A

Can you tell me what you did yesterday and whether you enjoyed it?

Exercise B

Can you tell me about the composition of your family?

Exercise C

Can you tell me about your pets?

7.2.6 *Explaining*

When explaining, the client allocates part of their attention capacity to memory, part to focus on the listener, and part to language formulation. As a result, less attention capacity remains for adjusting the speaking and articulatory rate to the linguistic demands of the exercise. To ensure the listener's attention, the client's story must align with the listener's prior knowledge and interest.

Exercise A

The speech therapist asks the client to explain the functional procedures for operating machines. It is essential to mention all the steps in the procedures.

Exercise B

The speech therapist asks the client to describe details of graduation at school. A higher level of complexity is expected.

Exercise C

The speech therapist asks a child or a young person with cluttering to explain the steps and different functions of a game. When the game is visible, the child/young person will present greater depth in explaining.

7.2.7   *Associative storytelling*

In the preceding exercises, the speech therapist only asked the client to describe what they observed or did. In this next level of language complexity, the speech therapist asks the client to present new ideas. In associative and creative storytelling, part of the client's attention capacity is used for memory, part to focus on the listener, part on suggesting creative ideas, and part on language formulation, so that all in all, there is little attention capacity left for the adjustment of the speaking and articulatory rate to the linguistic demands of this exercise.

Exercise A

Ask the client to explain what one does with a particular object. Then ask the client to elaborate on the explanation with, for example: 'You could also . . .,' or: 'If you change this, it's also possible to . . .'

Exercise B

The speech therapist can ask the client to describe new ideas (as in Exercise A) and explain why they would or would not be practical, or what is necessary to accomplish each new idea.

7.2.8   *Level 1–7, focusing on abstract concepts*

Using concrete words (high frequency) in the exercises is much easier than doing these exercises with abstract words (low frequency), such as 'disappointment,' 'vague,' 'impossible,' etc. The rate with which the word and the associated statement are selected certainly plays a role. Low-frequency words have a longer retrieval time than high-frequency words and expressions. The clients with cluttering speak fast and need help controlling this speed, especially since retrieving the words and sentence constructions takes longer for them.

Processing abstract words also requires additional effort from the listener, so the clients must really focus on the listener's perspective to know if their message is understood correctly.

What is word retrieval?

The terms 'word retrieval' and 'word finding' refer to the process of mentally identifying and then producing the word or words needed to express a thought or to name an object. Word finding is one of many types of information retrieval. Because words have two very different storage systems in the brain (one semantic and one phonological; see below), word retrieval depends on the development of both systems.

Semantic storage system (storage of meanings)

The meanings of words are stored in the brain as many circuits and systems of connections between nerve cells. These connections correspond to word associations. When a person is asked, for example, 'What is carp?', she may answer, 'A carp is a fish (category). Like all fish, they swim and breathe underwater (actions); they are not used for food (they taste like mud) but only for watching to (use/function); they have barbels —two short ones on the upper lip and two long ones in the corners of the mouth, and a long dorsal fin with very strong first fins. The fish can grow up to 47 inches in length; they are silvery and wide; and they weigh anywhere between 0.5 and 4 kilograms (attributes). In large sand extraction ponds with an area of more than 20 hectares, it is usually deeper than 32 feet (location). When I think of carp, I think of tough men with pictures of the giant carp they caught (idiosyncratic associations).'

The specific details aren't that important here; this is about the realization that word meaning is a collection of organized associations that correspond to large numbers of neural connections in the brain.

Phonological storage system

To say a word, we also need to know which sounds are needed to form the word. These sounds and their organization are stored in the brain's phonological storage system — again, a series of nerve cell connections, but this time not as extensive in the brain. The previous two storage systems must work to harmoniously support work retrieval quickly, smoothly, and effortlessly. The speed of word-finding depends on how frequently the word and its associations are used. High-frequency words are words used often in everyday life and thus frequently appear in ordinary conversations. Low-frequency words are words that are only used in certain situations. Often the phonological coding of these low-frequency words has yet to take place. In contrast, high-frequency words are spoken from current motor programs.

7.2.9 Discussing

Effectively performing complex linguistic tasks, such as arguing, advocating, defending, and reasoning, requires more effort and skill. The client must make several arguments to be convincing. Explaining why the client makes certain choices requires strong language formulation skills. If the client does not have these skills, the complexity of the exercise will affect the client's fluency or intelligibility.

Exercise A

The speech therapist asks the client to argue and reason on non-emotional topics. The speech therapist asks, for example: "Can you explain to me what you would change if you could be the President of the United States?"

Exercise B

The speech therapist chooses to work with emotional topics, such as arguing whether it is a good idea to donate money to developing countries. This can be done, for example, by asking the client to explain why she is or is not willing to transfer money for a UNICEF cause.

7.2.10 Persuading

In the previous step, arguing, one does not need to be focused on the ideas or beliefs of the listener. In this last step of language formulation, persuading the client must take the listener's ideas and beliefs into account. The attention capacity here is thus divided between many variables of interpersonal communication.

Exercise A

Start persuading by speaking about non-emotional topics. The speech therapist can start with speech assignments such as "Give a speech in which you persuade the Secretary of Education to cancel the student debt of 25- to 35-year-olds." Before the client starts persuading, a few minutes of preparation time is necessary.

Exercise B

Young people with cluttering can be asked to prepare a speech for their parents in which they try to persuade their parents to adjust something in the house rules to the young person's wishes.

Exercise C

Once persuading with non-emotional topics has been practiced, a speech therapist can choose to work with emotional topics. For example, ask the client to argue whether it is a good idea to make it mandatory for a therapist to volunteer for the chronically ill or elderly.

7.3   Speech rate reduction

Clients are barely able to adjust their speech rate to the linguistic demands of the moment. Or, as Ward stated (2018, p. 393): "If that internal clock is running at the wrong speed, is there anything that can reset it?" While clients can be taught how to slow down their speech rate, it takes an excessive attention capacity to achieve this goal, as most clients cannot automatize speech rate reduction. An attempt to do so requires a conscious decision or resolve, almost like the decision to learn a second language. A distraction can interfere with clients' attempts to practice their skills to the point where another conscious commitment must be made to resume working on the speech rate.

Ways to reduce speaking and articulatory rate:

- Audio feedback
- Audio-visual feedback
- Extension of pauses
- Syllable tapping
- Delayed articulation
- Feeling the movement of the articulators (kinesthetic feedback)
- Reading by breaking sentences into meaningful segments with slashes
- Exaggerated rhythm
- Exaggerated melody patterns

As shown in Figure 7.1, an adjustment of the speaking or articulatory rate influences several communicative components: Shared eye contact, the

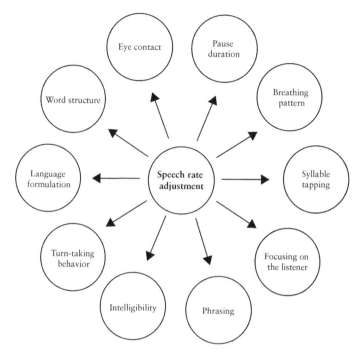

Figure 7.1 Effect of speech rate adjustment on communication behavior

pause duration, the breathing pattern, focusing on the listener, phrasing, intelligibility, turn-taking behavior, language formulation, and the word structure. Reducing the speech rate probably has a positive effect on other aspects of communication.

The methods that speech therapists choose to reduce the articulatory rate of their clients are determined by the skills and interests of the client and the linguistic context of the client's profession. Speech therapists determine the highest articulatory rate at which the client is still fluent and intelligible. Clients should not be asked to speak at the mean articulatory rate of the general population (5.0 SPS). If a client is fluent and intelligible at a rate between 6.5 and 7.5 SPS, that rate should be taken as a reference point. The speech therapist must maintain a rate margin of 1.0 SPS between the previously mentioned lowest and highest rates. In this case, the highest rate at which the client is still fluent and intelligible is 7.5 SPS, so the speech therapist aims for 7.5–1.0 = 6.5 as the lowest benchmark. A speech therapist should strive to ensure that fluent and intelligible speech is produced with a natural melody. An improved speech rate positively affects almost all symptoms of cluttering. Long-term control of the MAR in cluttering is possible by means of therapy targeting focused speech (Wiele & Zückner, 2019).

> The rate margin for each individual client will differ for every language complexity level.

7.4   Audio-visual feedback training (AVF)

Van Zaalen (2009) developed AVF training to help PWC improve their poor symptom awareness. PWC typically do not realize they have speech problems, so they believe their speech is understandable, fluent, and intelligible. But how do they not realize that their speech rate is too fast? Cluttering can be likened to driving race cars through a city, like Dubai, which is unfamiliar to the person with cluttering. Theoretically, it is possible to do this without damage, but this would require drivers to monitor their speed throughout the journey (brake), and that, likely, means that they will not be able to see and respond to all traffic signs along the road, nor to have a relaxed conversation with friends sitting in the passenger seats. How can these drivers be trained in their driving skills? Trainers would record the ride, play back the recording, discuss the traffic rules that need to be followed, plan improvements, and illustrate how these improvements can be made. Drivers retrained in this way will carry out any future attempt within the same general circumstances in a much more controlled manner. However, this occurs only if trainers take the time to acknowledge what has been done correctly and make drivers aware of what they did to make it right. This contrasts with the example of a coach who only points out the mistakes of a young, talented football player. After a while, this football player is fully aware of everything he is doing wrong, but in the meantime, he has no idea what to do to correct his mistakes, how to implement these corrections, and whether he can make the corrections.

Positive feedback is essential for AVF training. For example, while recording, the speech therapist can highlight the successful speech segments. Then, when playing this segment for the client, the speech therapist might comment, "Listen, this is very clear. We can see all the syllables on the screen, and every syllable of the word is audible and sounds natural. Let's listen again because it is very good. This is what we were aiming for. Let's measure your articulatory rate to have an idea of the rate at which you can be understood."

7.4.1   Rationale for the AVF training

As noted earlier, clients are often unaware of speech distortions when they occur. The fact that clinicians mention that according to PRAAT a client's speech is too fast, disfluent, or unintelligible is often not internalized in a way necessary for treatment (See the four-component model of cluttering in Chapter 6, Section 6.4). When listening to and watching the client's speech repeatedly, combined with analyzing rate, fluency, pause placement, and duration, the client observes and hears what a listener sees and hears. Instead of arguing that the rate is too high or that the speech is disfluent, in AVF training, speech is assessed by an analysis using PRAAT software. Such an approach is not based on a subjective opinion but on objective analysis. As a result of this analysis, the figures speak for themselves, as illustrated in the example below.

Without AVF-training

SLP: You've told me a story. What do you think of your speech rate?
Client: Well, I think it was okay.
SLP: I disagree.

Or:

Client: Oh, maybe it was a little too fast?
SLP: Glad you agree. Now for the next step . . .

Or:

Client: Well, it was slower than usual.
SLP: Then maybe you should listen more carefully.

With AVF training

SLP: You've told me a story. How about your speech rate?
Client: I think it was okay.
SLP: So, you think you're within the agreed rate range of . . . SPS?
Client: Yes, I think so.
SLP: Let's measure it.

After measuring:

SLP: We measured 2.0 SPS more than we agreed. What does that mean?
PWC: Oops, I spoke faster than I thought.
SLP: Okay, let's listen again and see what effect your speech rate had on your speech quality.

Without AVF training, there is a real risk that the speech therapist and the clients will not achieve sufficient progress in rate adjustment. After all, the perception of rate is influenced by subjective aspects such as the level of noise, the energy level of the listener, and the topic of conversation. For cluttering therapy to be efficient and effective long-term, objective measurements via PRAAT are necessary (Ward, 2018; Van Zaalen & Reichel, 2014).

After several sessions of AVF training, clients realize that they speak too fast, are disfluent, or need to be more intelligible. By playing and viewing their speech on the screen, the internal locus of control of the clients grows in terms of objectively analyzing their speech rate, disfluencies, and/or poor intelligibility. Showing the speech on the screen also provides the space needed to process any confrontational feedback. This distance is caused by the fact that there is often less direct eye contact between the speech therapist and a client during the analysis of speech via PRAAT.

The AVF training is more effective when longer recordings are used. The longer recordings (more than two minutes) prevent clients from reacting based on their memories of what they intended to say. And as discussed earlier with the 40-second rule, the focus will show the highest likelihood of the rate adjustment in the first 30 to 40 seconds, while the period after that shows the degree of automatization.

Once clients become aware of their speech disturbances, AVF training shifts focus from disfluency or impaired intelligibility to the moments of appropriate pauses or to a normal speech rate. After making appropriate pauses, clients' chances of the next sentence being fluent are much higher. Speech therapists should look for adequately long pauses. When a pause is detected with a duration of 0.5 to 1.0 seconds, the speech therapist should listen to determine whether the next phrase is indeed fluent or intelligible. By focusing on moments of success in this way, speech therapists can help their clients to build better speech control and increase their confidence in future successes. The clients learn what they can do to change their speech and how it sounds, looks, and feels when their speech is accurate, fluent, and intelligible. Positive audio feedback can be given in several ways: through a mobile phone recorder option, PRAAT software, Goldwave, Audacity, a WhisperPhone, or headphones with a microphone.

7.4.2   Subgoals for identification within AVF training

In AVF training, various aspects of speech, such as rate, fluency, pauses, melody, and loudness, are practiced. This leads to the following subgoals of the identification stage of treatment, which may or may not be implemented depending on the subtype of cluttering.

For syntactic cluttering

Subgoal 1: The client will be able to identify moments of fluent and disfluent speech in recordings of spontaneous speech with at least 80 percent accuracy.

Subgoal 2: The client will be able to identify interjections in recordings of spontaneous speech with at least 80 percent accuracy.

For both syntactic and phonological cluttering

Subgoal 3: The client will be able to identify the number and duration of pauses in recordings of spontaneous speech with at least 80 percent accuracy (both between phrases and between speakers). A pause, whether between speakers or phrases, lasts from at least 0.5 seconds to 1.0 seconds.

In phonological cluttering

Subgoal 4: The client will be able to identify the moments of intelligibility in recordings of spontaneous speech with at least 80 percent accuracy.

Subgoal 5: The client will be able to identify the moments of (melodic) monotony in recordings of spontaneous speech with at least 80 percent accuracy.

Subgoal 6: The client will be able to identify the moments of normal and excessive loudness in recordings of spontaneous speech with at least 80 percent accuracy.

7.4.3   Steps in the AVF training

Speech therapists can complete the following steps:

1. Determine the purpose of the recording exercises.
2. Determine how many 'errors' are considered acceptable.
3. Record the message with a digital audio recording system (software such as PRAAT, Audacity, or Goldwave is available as freeware) and save it as a *.wav file.
4. Write down the time of significant episodes on a piece of paper while recording.
5. Open the recorded file in PRAAT software.
6. Play a segment (maximum of 20 seconds) in which the goal set for the client has been achieved.
7. Ask the client to pay attention to specific aspects of speech production; for example: "Can you hear all the syllables in this piece?" or "Listen and count the number of 'uhs.'"
8. Measure and discuss the results.
9. Repeat steps 7 and 8 with a fragment that did not go well.
10. Repeat the exercise and compare the results of the first recording with the results of the second recording.
11. Schedule a practice assignment.

7.5   The treatment plan for syntactic cluttering

In syntactic cluttering, insufficient time is available for retrieving the word from the lexicon or for grammatical encoding. As a result, the client produces an excessive number of typical disfluencies. There are three factors essential to realize:

- The client produces an excessive number of typical disfluencies at a higher rate because insufficient time is available for the formulation phase.
- The client has no grammatical encoding problems, but revisions and phrase repetitions are used too fast to gain time.
- Pauses can increase the time available for formulation.

The four steps for the treatment of syntactic cluttering include:

1. Identification of disfluencies (see Section 7.5.1) and of interjections (7.5.2)
2. Identification of pauses and pause duration (7.5.3)
3. Speech rate adjustment (7.5.4)
4. Working on language formulation and story structure skills (7.5.5)

Cluttering therapy is often performed within a short time. The first two steps can enhance the client's communication skills, paving the way for steps 3 and 4; however, all steps are discussed in detail below.

7.5.1   *Identification of disfluencies*

Typical disfluencies are not consciously perceived by a speaker. After all, there is no tension or direct disruption of speech because of normal disfluencies. The way to familiarize the client with typical disfluencies is through AVF training. Therefore, follow the steps described in Section 7.4.3.

  Goal a: The client will be able to identify the moments of fluent and disfluent speech in recordings of spontaneous speech with at least 80 percent accuracy. After achieving this goal at all levels of language complexity, the client can move on to the next step, as described in Section 7.5.2. At the same time, the client can work on the second goal of this segment, goal **b**.

  Goal b: the client will be able to exhibit up to 10 percent of typical disfluencies to communicate within a level of language complexity with at least 80 percent of the recordings. Again, once the goal is achieved at a certain level of language complexity, the client can switch to practicing at the next level of language complexity. This approach to working within language complexity levels is consistent across all steps described in Sections 7.5 and 7.6.

Exercise A

Ask the client to share an experience and record it in PRAAT. At the end of the recording, ensure it is saved to the speech therapist's computer before

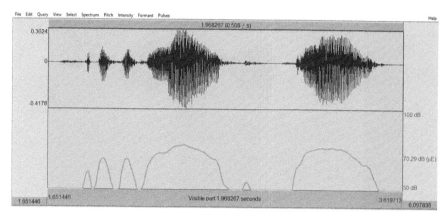

Figure 7.2 Representation of atypical disfluencies via PRAAT in the sentence "If I did, well well . . ." The repetition is visible in an almost exact copy of the production of the previous word.

importing it into PRAAT. When listening back, the speech therapist should choose a piece where the PWC repeats a word or phrase several times. Play this short segment multiple times and ask the client what stands out to them. Repeat a few times until the speech therapist observes a reaction from the client. The client is advised to make a new recording and subsequently to play a segment with disfluent speech. When the client plays the following piece and the speech therapist will say, "Hey, in this sentence, you only say all the words once, so you can do it without the repetitions." Then the speech therapist will suggest to the client to make another attempt. Each subsequent attempt will contain fewer disfluencies due to the client's added focus.

Exercise B

This exercise is similar to Exercise A but involves a more complex language level.

7.5.2 *Identification of interjections*

After identifying disfluencies, the topics of auditory perception and auditory discrimination for pinpointing interruptions should be discussed. This discussion should occur not only during sessions but also outside the therapy room. Clients with syntactic cluttering use an excessive number of interjections, such as "um," "you know," "actually," and "by the way," because their speech rate does not align with their language formulation (see Figure 7.3). In most cases, these interjections help clients to gain time for language formulation (including word finding). Identification of interjections makes clients aware of their difficulties in linguistic planning.

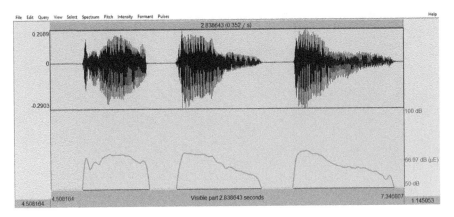

Figure 7.3 The /uh/ and the /um/ and the /ummm/ as they are identified in PRAAT

In addition, frequent use of interjections can adversely affect the comprehensibility and intelligibility of the message.

Note: It is not advisable to ask a client to count the number of interjections used by a speech therapist during a session. To do so would be too distracting for the client.

Exercise A

The speech therapist asks the client to observe other speakers use interjections several times. It is preferable to do this exercise while watching the news on television or listening on the radio. Practicing in this way does not disrupt communication between speakers and their environment. It is important to specify the duration and frequency with which the client should perform this exercise. The speech therapist also explains to the client how to process the data that is observed. Clients must write down, for example, how many interjections were present while listening to the news in the first five minutes.

Exercise B

As with many identification exercises, the speech therapist can ask the client to record phone calls or calls in Teams/Zoom/Webex and then listen to them. Remember, if the client records conversations, permission must first be obtained from the speaker. It might be wise to briefly explain the purpose and usage of the recording. Usually, speakers respond positively to such requests for permission.

Exercise C

Ask all family members to place a token "on the table" or "in a tray" or a plate or someplace else in front of them whenever they hear an "uhm" during a meal. Think of it as a funny identification game, just as you probably know the game "don't say yes, don't say no." You can make it more challenging for each other by asking questions about which issues need to be named or argued. The person who has collected the fewest number of tokens for "uhms" at the end of the meal does not have to wash dishes or clean the dishwasher.

7.5.3   Identification of pauses and pause duration

Example of working on pause duration within conversations in AVF training

"Let's look for a good pause . . . I hear and see a pause here and I think it's long enough . . . Let's measure it for a moment . . . Yes . . . This pause is 0.7 seconds . . . That will certainly influence the quality of the next sentence . . . I think this sentence will be fluent and intelligible . . . Let's listen for a moment . . . (listen) . . . What do you hear? . . . Fluent and intelligible! So, if you make a good pause, the next sentence will in all probability be fluent and intelligible. Good job."

A sample requires more than one pause. Speech therapists should ideally ask a client to measure five pauses within a two-minute recording and write down the duration of the pause in an Excel or Access table. Speech therapists must ensure that the client makes pauses between sentences or phrases and not within a phrase. The speech therapist instructs the client to take five measurements from a recording twice daily for their practice assignments. The client will assign a color to each range; for example, green when reaching the goal (for example, 0.5–1.0 seconds); orange when approaching the goal (for example, 0.3–0.49 seconds); and red when not coming close to the goal (for example 0–0.29 seconds). An example of this is given in Table 6.2 in Chapter 6. Experience shows that the comment, "See? You can already make appropriate pauses, but you still must learn to do that more often," has a positive impact on most clients, especially when introduced early in therapy.

Figure 7.4 represents a sentence followed by a 0.874690-second pause (highlighted in gray here). Figure 7.5 shows a pause of 0.676767 seconds in the middle of a sentence. It should be clear that PRAAT does not distinguish between a compound sentence and two simple sentences. PRAAT indicates the intensity of the sound information, and if no energy is observed in both the sound string (upper black waves) and the analysis (bottom gray line), there is a pause. By clicking on the gray bar at the bottom of the selected segment, you can play this piece for analysis.

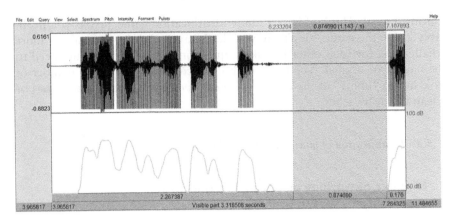

Figure 7.4 Selection of a pause, with a pause duration of 0.874690 seconds using PRAAT in a time frame of 3.318508 seconds

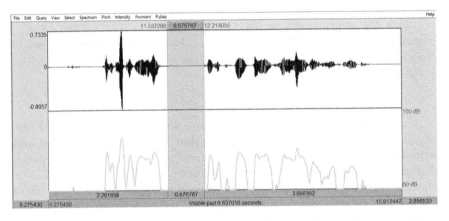

Figure 7.5 Pause selection, with a pause duration of 0.676767 seconds in a time frame of 6.637016 seconds

Note: When visually comparing the segments from different attempts, note that Figure 7.4 only displays 3.3 seconds of recording, while Figure 7.5 shows 6.6 seconds. Therefore, always take measurements instead of estimating.

7.5.4　*Adjustment of the speech rate*

Section 7.3 described the need, potential, and effects of speech rate reduction. The following exercises focus mainly on clients with syntactic cluttering as covered in Section 7.5.

> The human brain can process an average of 5.0 SPS.

Exercise A

A high speech rate can also be temporarily reduced by using delayed auditory feedback (DAF), frequency altered auditory feedback (FAF) or heightened auditory feedback (HAF). Using these feedback options, speech can be perceived as delayed (DAF), changed in pitch (FAF), or louder (HAF) while using headphones. Clients are directed to use a lower/higher pitch, speak louder, or delay their speech. If they focus more on their speech production, their rate will be significantly slowed down, resulting in temporarily improved speech. There is no empirical support for using DAF or FAF in cluttering. Most clients indicate that they find speaking under DAF or FAF conditions annoying. DAF/FAF software can be downloaded as Speech Monitor (Arenas, 2014).

In clinical practice, HAF appears to apply to everyone and can be very effective for PWC. PWC respond neutrally to the sound generated from HAF. Speech therapists are advised to use HAF, which can be done using a WhisperPhone, headphones with a microphone, sound-dampening headphones for construction workers, DAF software (where the delay is set to 0), or by having the PWC cover their ears with their hands. It is also recommended that speech therapists use HAF when testing the reading skills of children and adolescents. Choosing HAF for phone calls can produce positive effects for some PWC. Many clients with cluttering are unaware of a change at HAF, but internal and external monitoring work becomes a lot better because it provides better feedback.

Exercise B

The speech therapist can also provide direct feedback to clients by showing them a sign with a green and an orange side. In a conversation with clients, the speech therapist can show them the green side of the board if their speech rate is within acceptable limits, and they speak fluently or intelligibly. When clients start using telescoping or word and/or sentence repetitions, the speech therapist can warn them of their mistakes by using the orange side of the sign. The advantage of this color indicator approach is that every time the speech therapist shows a color, the client must interpret the meaning of the color and act accordingly. Practice shows that after using this rate indicator, clients began to anticipate the orange indicator in a few conversations and correct themselves even before the speech therapist could turn on the indicator – A sign that the auditory feedback loop of the client is doing its important job.

Exercise C

To make clients aware of their high rate of speech, the speech therapist imposes a "speeding fine" (St. Louis et al., 2003). This fine can take the form of a token on a table, a yellow card, or an additional practice request. A "too high rate" indicates the presence of frequent disfluencies or a higher number of them than usual.

Exercise D

The speech therapist instructs clients to set a speech rate goal before narrating a story for recording with PRAAT. Next, clients are asked to guess their speech rate: Above, below, or within the limits of the goal they set for their speech rate. The speech therapist and clients check this by measuring the speech rate. The speech therapist records all data in an Excel or Access file and points out the effect of the articulatory rate on comprehensibility and the number of disfluencies.

7.5.5   *Language formulation and storytelling structure*

Even though language disorders are not typical for cluttering, training in language formulation or story-telling skills is still beneficial for clients with cluttering. This applies to both children and adults.

Exercise A

With the "narrative tree," clients can develop their story structure skills. The speech therapist draws a trunk with five side branches and three offshoots per branch (see Figure 7.6). In the trunk, the speech therapist writes the subject. The client then determines the five themes that fit the main

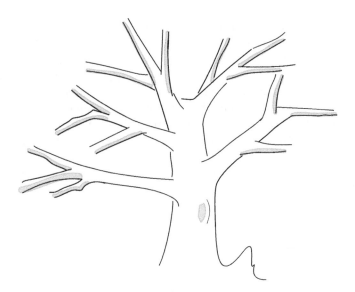

Figure 7.6 The storytelling tree

topic and places these themes (a word) in the side branches. The three off-shoots are then filled in for each theme. Only words are used when filling the tree. The formulation takes place during the tree's construction and the telling of the story. The client takes the drawings home and creates new ones as a home assignment.

Exercise B

In the "drawing comic strips" exercise, the listener draws an illustration for each sentence. A comic strip is created by placing all the drawings next to each other. Reviewing the comic strip with the client reveals areas with unclear statements or missing information. The comic strip can then be modified and/or supplemented. This creates a true story that can be taken home and told again. The chance of a successful experience in building a story structure is high.

7.6 The treatment plan for phonological cluttering

In phonological Cluttering, the phonological processes, motor planning, motor programming, and actual speech do not have sufficient time for completion. This is evident by clients' poor speech intelligibility, their very short pauses, pauses in linguistically inappropriate places, monotony, and disrupted speaking rhythm.

The five steps for the treatment of phonological cluttering are:

1. identification of impaired speech intelligibility (Section 7.6.1);
2. identification of pauses and pause duration (7.6.2);
3. improvement of auditory perception and syllable awareness (7.6.3);
4. speech rate adjustment (7.6.4);
5. improvement of prosody, speech rhythm, and melody (7.6.5).

In many cases of cluttering, the therapy time is limited, and Steps 1 and 2 strongly influence the aspects covered in Steps 3 to 5. Speech therapists should be aware that it may be important to complete only Steps 1 and 2, and it may not be necessary to go through Steps 3 through 5 with a client unless evaluation results show that the client needs to improve their speaking skills further.

7.6.1 *Identification of impaired speech intelligibility*

Feedback in running speech

During the session, the recorder will be stopped whenever an incorrect word or phrase is heard or seen. The client must accurately repeat an incorrect word in a controlled manner. If the client does not notice an incorrect word, the speech therapist will imitate the word in the way the client produced the word. Such an approach can be quite confrontational, so the speech therapist should clarify the goal of this imitation. It can be motivating for clients if they are able to produce the whole sentence correctly. The speech therapist's feedback is not effective enough if only the mispronounced words are corrected.

Feedback (directly) after production

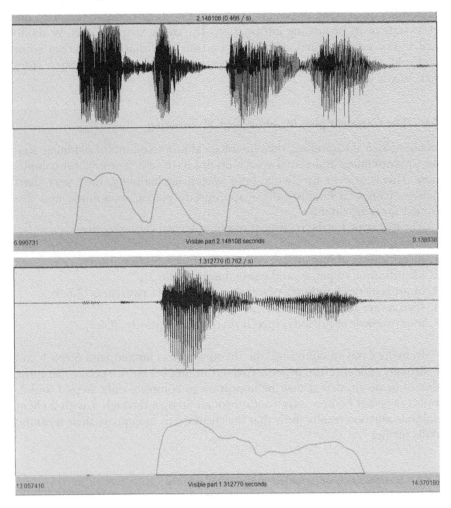

Figure 7.7 Identification of the syllables in the word 'intelligibility,' with on top clear syllable tapping and below with telescoping/coalescence.

Figure 7.7 shows two representations of the word 'intelligibility.' In the upper representation, the word is well articulated, with all the syllables included. In the second representation, not all syllables are accurately produced, resulting in reduced intelligibility.

Each peak refers to a vowel production. The higher the broken line, the louder the syllable is produced.

Practice word production

Exercise A

To practice at the word level, the client must repeat a difficult word five times, first with pauses between words and later without pauses. A client with intelligibility problems experiences the most difficulty with multisyllabic and low-frequency words. By repeating the words multiple times, the sequence of word retrieval, planning, and execution becomes more familiar. When practiced words are used more frequently, this sequence requires less focus to be performed correctly by clients. In addition, it is useful to praise clients multiple times in each session for controlled and intelligible word productions. By doing this, the speech therapist rewards the desired behavior.

Exercise B

When playing back and listening to digital recordings using PRAAT speech analysis software, a selected clip can be repeated as many times as necessary. Repetition increases the effect of direct feedback. Speech therapists ensure the fragment is long enough for the client to hear the intended productions. No additional word productions need to be played back.

Exercises for jaw-clamped speech/mumbling

Poor intelligibility can result from a jaw that is almost completely clammed shut, leading to mumbled speech due to minimal muscle or jaw activity. A limited jaw opening negatively affects intelligibility, when vowels are distorted, and consonants lose their precision. Such indistinct and mumbled speech can be addressed in therapy. Speech intelligibility is often improved by using speech rate reduction exercises. The effect of the insufficient jaw opening can be explained and assessed by using PRAAT.

Figure 7.8 shows that speech therapists can hardly detect jaw-clamped speech by using simple speech analysis via PRAAT. Even in the more complex analyses, which also display the formants and spectrum alongside loudness, the difference is hard to discern. It is recommended that the speech therapist selects the phrases and has them assessed by the clients.

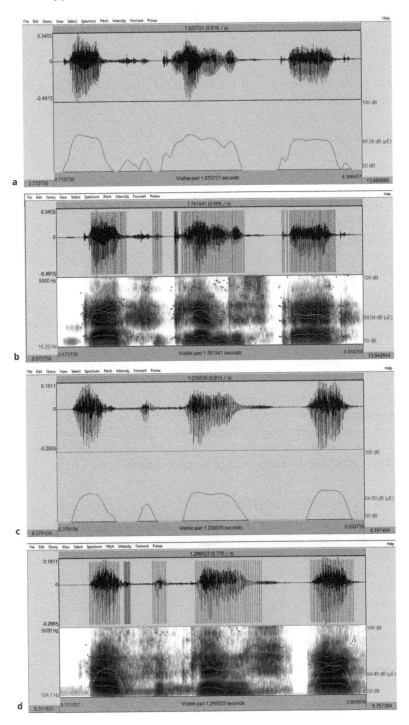

Figure 7.8 Display of syllable tapping and jaw-clamped speech in a simple (a+c) and a more complex representation (b+d)

Exercise A

Practicing in front of a mirror with word lists and sentences where the phoneme /a:/ occurs regularly can be beneficial. It might also be helpful to "measure" the degree of the jaw opening with fingers positioned horizontally.

Exercise B

The client reads rap lyrics aloud. Following that, the client can place a cork between their teeth and read the text again. Finally, the client can read the same text for a third time without the cork. Next, the client is asked to think about the differences felt during speech production. Recordings of all three attempts are then played via PRAAT.

More techniques to increase monitoring skills can be found in Myers (2011).

7.6.2   *Identification of pauses and pause duration*

Pauses in speech are crucial for producing and understanding speech. To monitor speech at the sentence level, a speaker needs sufficient pause time between sentences. Pauses between sentences create normal breathing patterns. The appropriate pause provides enough time to plan the structure of a new production. Pauses are also necessary for listeners' speech understanding. If pauses are too short, listeners might think the speaker has stopped talking. Additionally, when pauses are brief, listeners may require more time to process what is said. Both types of pause problems can lead to miscommunication. Pause duration correlates with the speech rate: the faster the speech, the shorter the pauses.

It is advisable to use PRAAT when addressing pauses. How PRAAT can be used when working on the speech rate is explained and presented in detail in Section 7.5.3; Table 6.2 shows how to display the pause duration.

Clients have a significant benefit in practicing appropriate pause lengths only if they have an opportunity to listen to the effect of exercises on their intelligibility. It is recommended that speech therapists use audiovisual feedback, check whether the pauses in the recordings are of sufficient duration, and listen to the phrase or clause following the pause being measured.

Additional visualization options for pauses

Silent blocks can be visualized using the spectrogram patterns in a PRAAT analysis. In contrast to regular phrasing, additional pauses can be visualized using the 'pulses.' It is normal to have four pulse blocks within 20 seconds (i.e., four clauses in 20 seconds).

Exercise A

The speech therapist instructs the client to pause for 0.5–1.0 seconds. The speech therapist creates a table. After recording, pauses are measured with PRAAT. Pauses of 0.0–0.2 seconds should be drawn in red. Pauses of 0.21–0.50 seconds are drawn in orange. Pauses of 0.5–1.0 seconds are drawn in green. Red means "unacceptable," orange means "almost succeeded," and green means "succeeded." Choose "almost succeeded," because if a speech therapist tells the client that orange means "not good," chances are that almost all attempts will be unsuccessful, and this can be very discouraging to the client. By utilizing these windows of opportunity, the speech therapist aims to increase the chances for successful productions: "Today, 15 out of 20 were in the 'almost succeeded' category. You also had 2 in the green group. Wow! I'm very proud." This approach is very motivational for everyone involved.

Exercise B

Places to pause can be identified using a text where the pauses have been removed. In this exercise, the client indicates where a small pause should separate words or phrases.

By reading texts or sentences aloud, where the speech therapist has deliberately inserted pauses in inappropriate places, the client can understand the importance of pause placement and learns how incorrect pauses affect comprehension of the text.

Exercise C

For an experienced client, quotes or short jokes can serve as good material for practice.

7.6.3   *Improvement of auditory perception and syllable awareness.*

Training in self-awareness is essential when working on the speech production of PWC. The main focus of speech production will be on the articulatory rate. The running of syllables into each other (telescoping or coalescence) is a characteristic of phonological cluttering and occurs due to the poor adjustment of the articulatory rate. Syllable awareness improves if clients allocate sufficient time for each syllable.

Exercise A

Syllable awareness can be facilitated by using syllable tapping or counting the syllables on the fingers. Speech therapists can ask their clients to determine the number of syllables in multisyllabic words. By the client's comparing the number of syllables with those of the speech therapist, the client gains insight into the accuracy of their syllable calculation.

Exercise B

In a game, use the number of syllables in the word given by the child instead of rolling a die.

Exercise C

Use "walking syllables." The longer the words, the faster you reach the target location. If you take incorrect steps, you will return.

Exercise D

Another way to enhance auditory perception is by developing an understanding of word- and sentence duration. PWC with phonological cluttering are often known for their poor time planning. For example, they can only allot enough time to produce three syllables when five syllables need to be produced. One way to address this telescoping is to repeat words, phrases, or entire sentences during the pauses of an audio recording. This exercise can be performed as follows: The client reads a line from a short poem. They are silent as they listen to the sentence and then repeat the phrase in their mind. They then read the next word, sentence, or line. They continue reading the following lines in the same manner. After about five lines, the recording is played, and the text is set aside. During the pauses in the recording, the client repeats the word or phrase. Often the pauses turn out to be too short. This exercise is repeated until the client has developed a better awareness of word and syllable duration. This improved syllable duration awareness can also help the client to produce pauses with the correct duration. This exercise can be evaluated by the percentage of syllables accurately produced during the recorded pauses.

Exercise E

An effective but challenging exercise for encouraging monitoring outside of the therapy room is to create a transcription of the client's reading of a text or a phone call with poor speech intelligibility. A client with poor auditory perception is asked to write down what they think they heard or thought they were saying. Writing down words syllable by syllable enhances the client's understanding of their speaking behavior. This is similar to the transcription based on a language sample. Transcribing is more challenging and, therefore, more effective when done the next day. It takes some practice to be able to transcribe a client's own speech correctly. The client can start this exercise by transcribing a musical track. If a person can do that within a therapy session, transcribing a song or their recordings can be given as a next practice assignment. To simplify this exercise, the speech therapist can limit the number of recordings that need to be transcribed.

7.6.4 *Adjustment of the speech rate*

Section 7.3 provides a detailed description of the need, options, and effects of the speech rate reduction exercises. The following exercises in this area are mainly focused on the treatment of people with phonological cluttering (see Section 7.6).

Exercise A

The diagnostic exercise of counting backward can be assigned regularly as a home assignment during therapy. This exercise can serve as a warm-up and gradually be made more complex (for example 101 minus 3; 201 minus 4 or 502 minus 7).

Exercise B

One can learn to identify the articulatory rate by getting clients to compare rates that are too fast with rates that are normal, upon reviewing their own recordings. This exercise can be practiced effectively by using AVF training.

7.6.5 *Prosody, speech rhythm and melody*

Stress patterns, pauses, and intonation impact how easily a person's speech is understood when listened to. Many PWC speak monotonously which can be manifested in two ways: (1) they always speak at the same pitch, or (2) they follow the same melodic pattern. In monotonous speech, all words and syllables have roughly the same pitch. Some PWC speak with melodic monotony: All sentences have approximately the same intonation pattern (see Chapter 2, Section 2.2.6).

> Normally, a person's voice volume fluctuates in a sentence within a ten dB range. When the volume level of PWC drops more than ten dB within one sentence, it is considered a symptom of insufficient breath support. This symptom is called the night candle effect and can be observed in people with Parkinson's as well. (See Section 2.2.6.)

Prosody

In phonology, prosody pertains to the rhythm, stress, and intonation used when producing sentences or phrases. For example, prosody can provide more information about the speaker's emotional state but also show whether a sentence is intended as a comment or a question. Prosody can also indicate whether the speaker is tense, cheerful, serious, or ironic. Prosody primarily relates to the acoustics of the spoken language. Issues raised in this context include syllable length and duration, loudness, pitch, and the formants of the speech sounds. In sign language, prosody is mainly linked to the length, tension, and rhythm of gestures. In written language, however, prosody plays no role. To convey aspects of prosody in written form, punctuation (e.g., commas, quotation marks, and ellipses) and typographic accentuation can be used. Emoticons can serve this purpose as well.

Exercise A

A speech therapist can ask the client to read a story containing characters' conversations. Such stories show pauses between sentences.

Exercise B

A speech therapist can ask the client to read or retell a fairy tale.

Exercise C

Rap lyrics are ideal for practicing rhythm and melody. A speech therapist can ask the client to prepare a rap at home (it can be an existing text) and have them perform it during the next session.

Speech rhythm

Speech rate and speech rhythm are not synonyms (see Section 2.2.7). A change in the speech rate directly impacts the speech rhythm and vice versa. Depending on the client, the speech therapist must determine whether working on the speech rhythm should be given priority. Clients are often unaware that each word has its own duration and that not all syllables last the same length of time. If an unnatural speech rhythm is caused due to working with syllable tapping, it is recommended to focus the client's attention on improving her speech rhythm.

Exercise A

During exercises for speech rate reduction, attention can be paid to the speech rhythm. Focusing on pauses or stress patterns may be a good option if speech rhythm cannot be differentiated from speech rate.

Exercise B

Practicing rhythm can be combined with exercises that facilitate exaggerated facial expressions and mimicry.

Melody

Melody also contributes to the perception of the message. Melody can be visualized using the "Intensity" tab in PRAAT. A blue line is visible on the screen. If the difference between the highest and lowest score (measured in the peak) shows a difference of between 80/100–200 Hz within a time frame of ten seconds, then the melody range is considered normal. It is considered monotonous if the score is less than 80 Hz (male) or 100 Hz (female). Melodic monotony takes place when the same melody pattern is repeated for each sentence. (see Section 2.2.6.) The melody is not tied to the pronunciation.

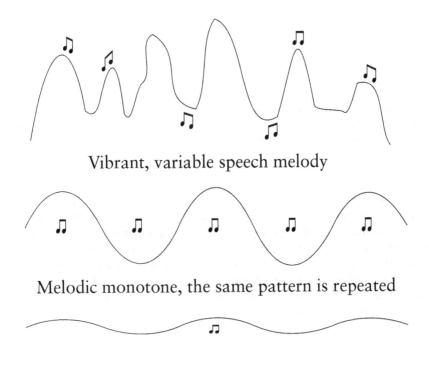

Vibrant, variable speech melody

Melodic monotone, the same pattern is repeated

Monotone, one tone, dull

Figure 7.9 Sentences with intonation patterns

Exercise A

Short jokes or excerpts from theater shows are particularly beneficial for practice with some PWC.

Exercise B

Reading interesting and significant news items online to friends, family, or colleagues ensures that PWC practice within a communicative context.

Exercise C

Practicing sentences in which the melody is visually represented (see Figure 7.9) can help clients who need clarification on the melody pattern to increase and decrease their speaking pitch.

7.7   The treatment plan for clients with combined cases of cluttering and stuttering

Before describing the priorities in treating cases of cluttering and stuttering, the background information on this topic will be provided. People who clutter and stutter (PWCS) generally find that cluttering is the primary disorder. The idea is that stuttering can develop based on cluttering, but not vice versa. This is also reinforced by the fact that when the speech rate of PWCS is slowed down, the stuttering decreases in frequency and intensity (Van Zaalen & Reichel, 2014). In such cases, treatment should first focus on cluttering. Only if the stuttering persists should the treatment also focus on stuttering. If the therapy leads to improvements, attention will increasingly be focused on cluttering. Even then, it is important to know whether the stuttering is accompanied by syntactic cluttering or by phonological cluttering. In the scientific literature from the last century, the treatment of cluttering-stuttering was often based on the personal judgment of researchers. No empirical studies have been conducted, and the published research often has not focused on specific exercises for people who exhibit both stuttering and a combination of syntactic or phonological subtypes of cluttering.

Myers and Bradley (1992) introduced a synergistic perspective in treating PWCS. This perspective integrates different approaches to treating clients that exhibit different symptoms, which interact, change, and affect each other in different ways. Addressing the complex interplay of these symptoms can be very challenging. Based on our clinical experience, it is recommended to prioritize the treatment of stuttering in children who have a high frequency of typical disfluencies. In adults with these symptoms, the cluttering component may be given priority when the stuttering-like disfluencies are produced with minimal tension, and when the individuals who stutter do not fear specific sounds or words. The rationale behind this is that people typically trip before they fall.

7.7.1   *Cluttering-stuttering: intervention strategies*

> You stumble before you fall, so if you do not stumble, you are much less likely to fall.

In this example, cluttering is represented as stumbling and stuttering as falling. If there are fewer or no cluttering episodes, there will likewise be fewer stuttering episodes in people with cluttering and stuttering. In cases where stuttering symptoms are addressed first, the cluttering symptoms should still receive similar attention. If not treated properly, the symptoms of cluttering will persist or worsen and can lead to a relapse of stuttering. Improving successful communication is a common goal for people with cluttering and stuttering. This goal encourages clients to independently select the techniques that work best for them at any specific moment of time in any speaking situation. Flexibility to adjust their techniques to any speaking situation requires automatic skills which contributes to the clients' confidence. To facilitate a faster transfer, the speech therapist should use those approaches that enhance the naturalness of speech the most. While practicing such techniques, PWCS must have a sense of safety and security not only in the motor aspect of speech but also in their mind during the planning stage of the message and during the formulating sentences stage. In other words, no discomfort should be anticipated; no fears should be experienced. Among the tools facilitating a sense of ease and comfort are phrasing, pseudo-stuttering, varying the length of the pauses at the phrase junctures, and modifying intonation and stress.

Once the sense of comfort is achieved, at the conversational level, PWCS learn to feel it and enjoy it. They they can then progress to use it in all settings. By becoming masters of such an approach and experiencing ease in communication, coupled with positive interactions, PWCS will transform their self-image and personal construct. It is crucial to praise and validate each PWCS whenever a goal is achieved. The experience of success and fulfillment of goals will bring them hope, pride, and courage to work on their remaining symptoms of cluttering through various activities, such as comparing different rates of speech, improving speech intelligibility, storytelling skills, word retrieval, and self-monitoring skills. Special attention should be paid to improving conversational skills (taking turns, staying on the topic, and considering the listeners' perspectives). Stuttering symptoms are likely to return if symptoms of cluttering are not addressed. Various strategies, like role-playing and counseling, should be used to address the cognitive, psychosocial, and emotional aspects of cluttering and stuttering disorders. Training in assertiveness, self-acceptance, positive self-image, and coping with negative stigma can be targeted to address a wide range of negative cognitions and emotions. To succeed in cluttering and stuttering intervention, speech therapists should go beyond the scope of the speech-language pathology field by intersecting advances across allied disciplines, such as cognitive-behavioral therapy, neural sciences, social sciences, positive psychology, mindfulness, emotional intelligence, and working alliance (Scaler Scott, Sønsterud, Reichel, 2022, Boyle, 2011; Mayer et al., 2000; Menzies et al., 2009; Ohman, 2000; Reichel, 2007, 2010; Reichel, St. Louis & Van Zaalen, 2013; Schneider, 2004; Shapiro, 2011; St. Louis, 2011; Weiss & Ramakrishna, 2006; Wilder, 1993).

7.7.2 *Priorities in the treatment of people with cluttering and stuttering*

When cluttering is accompanied by stuttering in adults, the specific symptoms of cluttering should be addressed first unless people have anxiety due to stuttering. St. Louis et al. (2003) and Van Zaalen and Winkelman (2014) argue that fluency-enhancing techniques, such as rhythmic speech with breathing exercises, can be used for this purpose. (See the counting backward exercises in Section 4.3.4). Once the PWC realize that their speaking has improved, their overall self-confidence will improve as well. The fear of stuttering is a persistent factor in cases of cluttering-stuttering. By increasing confidence in the speech of their clients with cluttering, speech therapists also help alleviate the fear of stuttering. A second reason to treat the cluttering component first is that if it is not addressed, the 'cluttering' symptoms will persist, potentially leading to a stuttering relapse. Weiss (1964) and Damsté (1984) have introduced this view of the treatment of cluttering-stuttering. A third reason to start with the cluttering component before treating the stuttering component is the initial lack of awareness of cluttering symptoms. Awareness of a person's speaking symptoms is necessary to achieve a permanent behavior change. Finally, when a person slows down the speech rate, as is necessary when addressing cluttering, it is much easier to apply the stuttering modification techniques.

In children with a combination of cluttering and stuttering, it is better to start therapy by devoting a few sessions to stuttering to prevent the development of anxiety. In these cases, working on stuttering is consistent with what children expect to address in therapy. Therefore, it helps to establish the right relationship between the child and the speech therapist. After a few sessions, if the relationship with the child is established, the speech therapist can make it clear that the symptoms of cluttering should be addressed as well.

7.8 Syllable tapping

Syllable tapping is an exercise that is not focused on communication. It can be compared to dry-land swimming. The next time the client speaks, she can rely on the skills she developed while practicing 'on dry land.' The advantage of syllable tapping is that it is very concrete, and the result can be immediately controlled with AVF. Moreover, the client often responds neutrally to syllable tapping. It is important to present the exercise to the client in a structured and clear manner. For this technique to succeed, the exercises must meet the SMART criteria, especially since speech can feel unnatural to clients who practice syllable tapping and because many of them need help to achieve their auditory monitoring goals.

The effect of syllable tapping exercises is influenced by the transfer to the next step, which can be taken when the previous step is completed correctly. The effect of syllable tapping also depends on the client's abilities, their compliance, and the frequency of the client's practice at home. Syllable tapping interrupts communication between the speech therapist and the client, forcing the client to speak at a slower rate.

As previously mentioned, syllable tapping is not recommended for clients with cluttering and stuttering. While tapping aims to generate change, for PWCS, syllable tapping might overemphasize speech production, potentially increasing muscle tension or leading to secondary behaviors. Stuttering can therefore be negatively affected by syllable tapping.

7.8.1   Steps in syllable tapping

Winkelman in Van Zaalen and Winkelman (2014) has achieved good results over the years with syllable tapping and described the steps of syllable tapping based on practice-based evidence.

Step 1

When reading a column of monosyllabic words, the client must tap on a table with a finger when pronouncing each word. No other body part should move with the rhythm, especially not the head.

Step 2

A column of two-syllable words can be tapped in a very fast manner. It is best to use the so-called spondees (two-syllable words with equal stress on both syllables), such as 'baseball,' 'maybe,' 'blackboard,' 'concept,' 'nervous,' etc. In words with unstressed syllables, such syllables are frequently deleted by clients.

Step 3

After practicing with two-syllable words, speech therapists transition to short sentences composed of two or three-syllable words. Keep in mind that clients will omit the unstressed syllables quite easily. It is, therefore, important to provide immediate feedback on these errors. At this stage, each tap should have the same duration, in a consistent rhythm. A metronome can be useful to help the client maintain the rhythm. If the client fails to identify syllables accurately, the speech therapist can suggest to the client to mark each syllable with a slash in the written text.

Exercise A

The speech therapist taps syllables in a sentence using the index finger and middle finger. The client imitates the tapping. The client taps the syllables of each word with a different hand. If this step is performed correctly, a transition to a standard text can be made. If the client corrects herself, the exercise is understood and syllable awareness increases.

Exercise B

The client taps the syllables when reading a text. A normal speech rhythm with normal rate changes should be practiced by tapping all syllables, including those without stress. An audio recording can show clients that their speech rate sounds natural.

Exercise C

Clients can also tap unnoticeably, specifically with their toes. This is a way of tapping that can be used well when speaking, standing up, or sitting behind a desk. It can help the client to begin a presentation, ask a question, or make a comment during a meeting.

Speech therapists should not presume that every adolescent or adult can accurately count syllables in words or the number of words in a sentence. A reliable method for the speech therapist to investigate whether the client can accurately count syllables in a line is to present a client with a sentence containing short, medium, and long words. For example, "My mom asked me to go to the nearby department store to buy us a delicious cheesecake."

7.9 Mindfulness

Ward (2018) has described mindfulness as a possible addition to existing cluttering therapy. He has indicated that a three-week mindfulness program significantly improved the speech of one person with cluttering. Of course, it is not possible to prove the intervention's effectiveness based on one success story. Still, the authors of this book often employ methods of inner peace, essential for facilitating the complex monitoring practiced by clients. Thus, they view the principles of Mindfulness-Based Cognitive Therapy (MBCT) as a potential basis for promoting inner peace in PWC.

The concept of mindfulness originates in many meditative, cultural, and philosophical traditions. While Buddhism offers extensive teachings on mindfulness principles and exercises, individuals can practice mindfulness without adhering to a specific philosophical, religious, or cultural tradition (Kabat-Zinn, 2000). Mindfulness involves "paying attention in a certain way, on purpose, in the present moment, and nonjudgmentally" (Kabat-Zinn, 1994, p. 4). It refers to continuously cultivating consciousness and conscious attention. The quality of consciousness sought in mindfulness exercises encompasses openness, curiosity, and a nonjudgmental attitude. The emphasis is placed on seeing and accepting things as they are without trying to change them.

As mentioned, mindfulness exercises and principles originate in many meditative and philosophical traditions. The recent surge of interest regarding mindfulness in therapeutic techniques can be attributed to the publication of some well-designed empirical evaluations of MBCT. The theoretical and empirical literature on therapeutic applications of mindfulness is growing. For instance, Oliva et al. (2021) explore the efficacy of mindfulness-based therapy on AD(H)D, considering its associated characteristics, clinical contexts, neurocognitive impairments, daily functions, and quality of life. They suggest that mindfulness-based interventions may be of added value to other effective interventions.

Mindfulness contrasts with the ordinary mental state of being "on auto-pilot." Mindfulness is not primarily goal-oriented, despite the exercise having certain secondary effects. While mindfulness can induce relaxation, its primary purpose is not a 'relaxation exercise.' It promotes non-judgmental awareness of the body and mind's state. It is therefore the appropriate exercise that can be implemented without any expectation of results, no matter how desirable those results may be.

Mindfulness can be cultivated through various techniques, all of which have a meditative component. In addition to formal mindfulness meditation (normally a sitting or lying meditation), these techniques include mindfulness of movement (with both yoga and mindful walking) and short periods of "mini meditation" throughout the day. This also encompasses the concept of everyday mindfulness; that is, remaining conscious in the present moment, even during seemingly routine tasks like brushing one's teeth.

The development of effective emotional regulation is critical to the success of PWC in various settings. These skills are especially important for PWC, who must learn to deal with diverse listeners daily. Research by Alahari (2017) suggests that mindfulness exercises contribute to the social-emotional competence and psychological well-being of teachers; possibly, mindfulness could also support PWC in better attuning themselves to their listeners. To investigate this suggestion, further scientific research will be needed.

During mindfulness exercises, practitioners aim to maintain focus on a particular point, often the sensations of their breathing. Strong attention skills are essential for self-regulation, and in turn, effective self-regulation is crucial for managing health problems like cluttering. Self-management requires not only attention but also 'thinking' in the form of complex cognitive functions, such as analysis and planning. Mindfulness training appears to improve the patient's attention and cognitive functions at a basic level. Attention involves multiple processes: focusing, recognizing, wandering, and refocusing. Different brain networks play a role in this (Van Burken et al., 2017). When the attention wanders from the breath, the patient will notice and let go of thoughts and feelings, and attention is returned to breathing (Alahari, 2017). This process is repeated every time attention wanders, simply paying attention to where the thought is wandering and accepting the wandering without passing judgments or elaborating on its implications.

The authors do not take a position as to whether mindfulness is effective for cluttering. However, any support that enables PWC to speak more consciously and enhances focused attention might be valuable, as long as it does not exhaust their attention capacity. This is why, as mentioned above, the authors have incorporated methods of inner peace in their treatment of cluttering.

7.10   In conclusion

This chapter outlines a cluttering therapy program incorporating various suggested and alternative exercises. Training in self-awareness is the highest priority. The new speaking pattern should be adopted automatically and effortlessly and should become the client's natural mode of communication. In cluttering therapy, frequent and brief home exercises are essential to facilitate gradual generalization to the new speech pattern in all communicative situations.

The authors hope that this book will contribute to the noble efforts of dedicated professionals by ending the neglect and misconceptions of cluttering, so that PWC may communicate effectively, and lead a vibrant and fulfilling life, with respect and acceptance by every individual in every societal community.

Appendices

Cluttering Assessment Battery

(van Zaalen, 2009)

Appendix	Title
A	Predictive Cluttering Inventory-Revised (PCI-r
B	Analysis of Spontaneous Speech, Reading, and Retelling
C	Mean Articulatory Rate
D	Retelling a Memorized Story: "The Wallet Story"
E	Screening Phonological Accuracy (SPA)
F	Oral-Motor Assessment Scale (OMAS)
G	Brief Cluttering and Stuttering Questionnaire (BCS)
H	Reading Text for Adult Readers
I	Speech Situation Checklist for Cluttering

Additional Appendices

Appendix	Title
J	Cluttering Statement
K	Personal Stories of People with Cluttering and Stuttering
L	Reading Passages

Appendix A
Predictive Cluttering Inventory-Revised (PCI-r)

Original by Daly and Cantrell (2006); revised version by Van Zaalen et al (2009).

Instructions to SLP

Ask the client to speak for 2–3 minutes about an experience during the holidays last year. This task is meant to be a monologue, rather than a dialogue. If the client starts to sum up, ask them to explain the rules of a sports activity or a certain procedure.

Please respond to each section below. Circle the number you believe is the most descriptive of this client's cluttering during the evaluation. Count the scores of the italic items in each section.

	5 Always	4 Almost always	3 Frequent	2 Sometimes	1 Almost never	0 Never
Section 1: Speech-motor						
1 *Lack of pauses between words and phrases*						
2 *Repetition of multi-syllablic words and phrases*						
3 *Irregular speech rate; speaks in spurts or bursts*						
4 *Telescopes or condenses words*						
5 *Initial loud voice trailing off to unintelligible murmur*						

	5 Always	4 Almost always	3 Frequent	2 Sometimes	1 Almost never	0 Never
6 *Oral diadochokinetic coordination below expected normed levels*						
7 *Rapid rate (tachylalia)*						
8 *Co-existence of excessive disfluencies and stuttering*						
9 *Speech rate progressively increases (festinating)*						
10 *Poor planning skills; misjudges effective use of time*						
Total italic items section 1						
11 Little or no excessive effort observed during disfluencies						
12 Poor planning skills for pauses (place and duration)						
13 Articulation errors						
Section 2: Language planning						
14 Disorganized language increases as topic becomes more complex						
15 Poor language formulation; poor story-telling; sequencing problems						
16 Language is disorganized; confused wording; word-finding problems						
17 Many revisions; interjections; filler words						

	5 *Always*	4 *Almost always*	3 *Frequent*	2 *Sometimes*	1 *Almost never*	0 *Never*
18 Inappropriate topic introduction, maintenance, or termination						
19 Improper linguistic structure; poor grammar; syntax errors						
20 Variable prosody; irregular melody or stress pattern						
Section 3: Attentiveness						
21 Does not recognize or respond to listener's visual or verbal feedback						
22 Does not repair or correct communication breakdowns						
23 Lack of awareness of own communication errors or problems						
24 Speech better under pressure (improves short-term with concentration)						
25 Distractible; poor concentration						
26 Attention span problems						
27 Seems to verbalize before adequate thought formulation						
28 Little or no anxiety regarding speaking; unconcerned						

	5 *Always*	4 *Almost always*	3 *Frequent*	2 *Sometimes*	1 *Almost never*	0 *Never*
Section 4: Motor planning (describe these symptoms compared to age level norms)						
29 Clumsy and uncoordinated; motor activities accelerated or impulsive						
30 Writing includes omission or transposition of letters, syllables, or words						
31 Poor motor control for writing (messy)						
32 Compulsive talker; verbose; tangential; word-finding problems						
33 Poor social communication skills; inappropriate turn-taking; interruptions						
Interpretation Section one: > 24 points in italic items → possible cluttering Section two: items provide information on linguistic component in cluttering Section three and four provide additional information about client's communicative skills						

Appendix B
Analysis of Spontaneous Speech, Reading and Retelling

Purpose

By means of the *Assessment Form for Analysis of Spontaneous Speech, Reading and Retelling*, clinicians will be able to get more knowledge about the normal and stuttering-like disfluencies and the ratio of disfluencies. The form is filled in for all three speech tasks seperately. A comparison of the results in the different speech tasks gives the clinician insight into the influence of linguistic complexity on speech output.

Assessment

The client will be asked to say something spontaneously, read a story, and retell a story. These assessment tasks will be audio and video recorded. When clinicians proceed to fill in the form, they should start at a random moment of speech. They differentiate between normal and stuttering-like disfluencies during the speech sample analysis. Clinicians should only count normal disfluencies. They should not count multisyllabic word repetitions, interjections and revisions (interjections and revisions are normal disfluencies).

Analysis and interpretation

The sentences the client produces will be scored based on the types of normal disfluencies.

Example						Summary
The client says: *I can't can't go on on holiday tomrow*						* 6 Stutter free words
I	can't	Go	On	Holiday	Tomorrow	* 2 Normal disfluencies
__	WR	__	WR	__	T	1 extra characteristic consistent with cluttering

Normal disfluencies (NDF)

Normal disfluencies can be categorized as follows:

word repetition (WR)	Repetition of a word in a relaxed manner in a calm rate.
part word repetition (PWR)	Repetition of a part of a word in a relaxed manner in a calm rate. Example: 'dif-different.'
interjection (Int.)	Insert a word or phrase which is inconsistent with the grammar or linguistic structure. Example: 'You know' or 'uuh.'
revision (Rev.)	A reformulation of an utterance. Example: 'I'm going, I went to school.'
phrase repetition (PR)	A repetition of a part of a sentence. Example: 'I went, I went, I went to school.'
Total number of normal disfluencies (NDF)	The total will be determined by the sum of the normal disfluencies mentioned above.

Stuttering-like disfluencies

Stuttering-like disfluencies can be categorized as follows:

tense word repetitions (tWR)	Repetition of a word in a tense manner in a rapid or dysrhythmic rate.
tense part-word repetitions (tPWR)	Repetition of a part of a word in a tense manner in a rapid or dysrhythmic rate. Example: 'dif-different.'
prolongations (Pro.)	The continuation of a sound at the articulation place. Example: 'ffffffffffffffish.'
blocks (Block)	The stream of breath stalls during the production of a sound. The sound can no longer be produced. This results in a very powerful production of the sound. Example: '......Book.'
Stuttering-like disfluencies (SDF)	The total will be determined by the sum of the stuttering-like disfluencies mentioned above.

Example						Summary
The client says: *I ca-ca-ca-can't go on on hhhhhhholiday tomorrow*						* 2 Stuttered words
I	can't	Go	On	Holiday	Tomorrow	* 1 Normal disfluency
—	/ tPWR	—	WR	/ Pro	T	* 1 extra characteristic consistent with cluttering

Interpretation

Normally people adjust their speech rate to more complex linguistic tasks and thereby prevent a higher frequency of disfluencies. If people are not able to adjust their speech rate to the complexity of the task, a more complex task will provoke more normal disfluencies.

See Assessment Form on next page.

Assessment Form: Percentage of Typical and Stuttering-like Disfluencies
Name:
Date:
Age:
Task: □ Spontaneous speech □ Retelling □ Reading

										Type	Number
										WR	
										pWR	
										PR	
										Int	
										Rev	
										TDF	
										tWR	
										PRO	
										Block	
										SDF	

Comments on secondary behavior
o   Visible:
o   Auditory:

Appendix C
Mean Articulatory Rate

Purpose

The assessment of the articulatory rate is crucial in determining whether the speaker has the obligatory symptom of an excessivley high and/or an excessively variable articulatory rate. Only in that case can cluttering be diagnosed.

Assessment

The articulatory rate will be determined by analyzing samples of speech from the audio or video recordings of spontaneous speech, reading and retelling.

Form for Assessment of Articulatory Rate			
Name:			
Date:			
Age:			
Measurement	Spontaneous speech sample	Retelling	Reading
1.			
2.			
3.			
4.			
5.			
Mean Articulatory Rate			
Variation within speech condition			
Variation between speech conditions			

Analysis

Five measurements of the articulatory rate will be taken randomly from each digital audio recording.

The articulatory rate measurements should be perfomed on at least 10 and at most 20 syllables of fluent speech. Utterances with nonfluent speech, pauses or
interjections should not be included in the analysis. These disturbances have unwanted effects on the reliability of the measurements.

The measurements will be performed by using the speech analysis software PRAAT (Boersma & Weenink, 2022).

Interpretation

Norms for the articulatory rate at different ages	Articulatory Rate variation (ARV)
Syllables per second (SPS) Mean Articulatory Rate spontaneous speech ○ Children > 5.2 SPS ○ Adolescents > 5.6 SPS ○ Adults > 5.4 SPS	Adequate rate variation: 1.0 < VAR < 3.3 SPS Cluttering: VAR < 1.0 between speech tasks and/or VAR > 3.3 SPS within speech task

If the variation within the same speech condition, between the highest and the lowest measurement, is higher than 3.3 SPS, the articulatory rate is considered to be too variable. If the variation between different speech conditions is 1.0 SPS or lower, then the variation is too rigid. So inadequate adjustment of the articulatory rate to the speech condition or language complexity is indicative of cluttering.

Appendix D

Retelling a memorized story

The Wallet Story

Purpose

While a client is retelling a memorized story, the clinician can observe to what extent the client is able to convey a message that someone else has already formulated.

Instruction

The clinician should tell the client: 'I will read you a story. After I have finished reading the story, please retell back to me the same story as completely as possible. I am not allowed to help you with it.'

The Wallet Story

It was a rainy day in November. A woman drove to the supermarket in her brand new car. She invited three girlfriends to dinner that night, and had promised them that she would prepare something Italian. That was her speciality. While she was shopping, her wallet fell from her pocketbook, but she did not notice it. Her shopping cart was already loaded. When she arrived at the cashier, she could not pay for her groceries. The cashier was willing to watch her shopping cart for a while. The woman put her groceries aside, and went home. The windshield wipers of her car moved rapidly from side to side. All the traffic lights she encountered were red, of course. She was terribly fed up! Just when she opened the door to her house, the phone started ringing. A little boy told her he had found her wallet. The woman was very relieved. The end.

Scoring form for the Wallet Story

(Van Zaalen, Wijnen, & Dejonckere 2009)

Main issues	Side issues	Story	Clients response	Syntax	DF
Name					
Date					
Age					
				Not	
				correct	
1		It was a rainy day in November.			
2		A woman drove to the supermarket in her brand new car.			
3		She invited three girlfriends to dinner that night,			
	1	and had promised them that she would prepare something Italian.			
	2	That was her speciality.			
4		While she was shopping,			
5		her wallet fell from her pocketbook,			
6		but she did not notice it.			
	3	Her shopping cart was already loaded.			
7		When she arrived at the cashier, she could not pay for her groceries.			
	4	The cashier was willing to watch her shopping cart for a while.			
	5	The woman put her groceries aside,			
8		and went home.			
	6	The windshield wipers of her car moved rapidly from side to side.			
	7	All the traffic lights she encountered were red, of course.			
	8	She was terribly fed up!			
9		Just when she opened the door to her house,			
10		the phone started ringing.			
11		A little boy told her			
12		he had found her wallet.			
	9	The woman was very relieved.			
13		That was the story.			

Of the 13 main issues the client retold . . . . . . main issues (almost) completely.

Of the 9 side issues the client retold . . . . . . side issues (almost) completely.

The proportion of main issues to side issues is . . . . . . : . . . .

Total number of grammatically correct sentences: . . . .

Total number of sentences with the incorrect use of structure: . . . .

Mistakes in linguistics: . . . .

Mistakes in syntax: . . . .

Of the 13 main issues the client retold . . . . . . main issues (almost) completely.

Of the 9 side issues the client retold . . . . . . side issues (almost) completely.

The proportion of main issues to side issues is . . . . . . : . . . . . .

Analysis

1. Transcribe the story told by the client.
2. Determine story components (main issues, side issues and noise).
3. Determine the correct use of syntax (% correct; % incorrect).
4. Determine type and percentage of dysfluencies and moments of telescoping/coalescense.

Appendix E
Screening Phonological Accuracy (SPA)

Purpose

This assessment can provide insight into speech-motor skills at the word level in test conditions. Of ten test words, only the three boldfaced words are analyzed as to being correct/incorrect productions and consistent/inconsistent (the three attempts are the same/or different). Mean articulatory rate is determined.

Instruction

The clinician should tell the client: 'Please look at these words for up to 5 seconds. Then I will cover the words and ask you to repeat the words 3 times in consecutive syllable strings, in a fast but still intelligible manner and without pauses.'

Words

Previously unpublished encounters – Distinctive sounds – Clinical management perspective – **Possible probabilities** – Epidemiological data – Screaming and shrieking audience – **Impracticable communicative implications** – Hierarchically organized behavior – Most favored nation clause – **Compromised alternative condemnation** – Frequently used devices – Delayed auditory feedback.

Scoring

The most important feature to observe is the consistency in the production of the sequence. In other words, whether production 1 is similar to production 2, and to production 3. If not, it indicates planning or phonological encoding problems.

Screening Phonological Accuracy
Dutch version: Van Zaalen, 2009
English version: Van Zaalen, Cook, Elings & Howell, 2011

Name:

Date:

Age:

Language:

Word strings	Correct	Incorrect	Consistent	Inconsistent	MAR
Possible probabilities					
Impracticable communicative implications					
Compromised alternative condemnation					

Interpretation
The person is able to produce correct and consistent word strings at a fast rate: not indicative of phonological cluttering.
The person is not able to produce correct and consistent word strings at a fast rate: indicative of phonological cluttering.

Appendix F
Oral-Motor Assessment Scale (OMAS)

Purpose

Van Zaalen et al. (2009b) found no correlation between accuracy, smooth flow, and rate scores in oral-motor control and speech-motor control at the word level. If it turns out that in the articulation screening the client makes more word structure errors than normal, the OMAS can be used to rule out weak oral-motor skills as the cause of word structure errors. The OMAS cannot be used as a differential diagnostic instrument for cluttering and other disorders of fluency.

Assessment

During this test, the following three syllable sets will be evaluated:

- puh
- tuhkuh
- puhtuhkuh

The clinician should model the syllable sets. The client must produce the sets at least ten times in a row, at a rapid rate. The assessment should be audio recorded and should be evaluated as to accuracy, equability and rate.

Analysis and interpretation

By means of the Norm Table, the scores can be interpreted and a determination can be made as to whether there are any oral-motor problems which cause word structure errors.

Scoring Form for the Oral-Motor Assessment Scale

Name:					
Date:					
Age:					
Syllable set	Correct	Incorrect	Consistent	Inconsistent	Mean Articulatory Rate
Pa Ta-Ka Pa-Ta-Ka					
Conclusion					

Analysis and interpretation

If the score deviates > 1.5 SD of the norm, it can be concluded that the oral - motor control is below the age-appropriate level. If a weak score on OMAS is accompanied by word structure errors or phonetic defects, then training of oral -motor skills is recommended.

Norm Table OMAS based on Riley (1985) & Van Zaalen (2009)						
	Age	Mean	- 0.5 sd	- 1.0 sd	- 1.5 sd	- 2.0 sd
Puh	8	2.1	2.3	2.5	2.7	2.8
	9	2.0	2.2	2.4	2.6	2.7
	10–11	1.8	2.0	2.2	2.4	2.5
	12	1.7	1.9	2.0	2.2	2.3
	13+	1.6	1.9	2.0	2.1	2.3
Tuhkuh	8	4.8	5.5	6.1	6.5	7.5
	9–10	4.4	5.0	5.5	6.0	6.6
	11–12	3.8	4.3	4.7	5.1	5.5
	13+	3.4	3.9	4.3	4.7	5.1
Puhtuhkuh	8	8.3	9.3	10.3	11.3	12.3
	9	7.7	8.7	9.7	10.7	11.7
	10	7.1	7.9	8.6	9.4	10.1
	11–12	6.5	7.2	8.0	7.9	9.6
	13+	5.7	6.4	7.2	8.0	8.7

Appendix G
Brief Cluttering and Stuttering Questionnaire (BCSQ)

Purpose

When clients present with cluttering and stuttering at the same time, their personal experiences influence how the two disorders impact on communication skills, fear and avoidance behavior. Although some symptoms are easier to treat in therapy than others, priorities in treatment should be based on the clients' complaints. In other words, zoom in to the complaints and zoom out to the client. Responses to this brief questionnaire provide insights into the impact of stuttering and cluttering on the lives of clients.

Instructions

When clinicians have clients complete the questionnaire, the interview should be flexible enough to allow clients to elaborate on one question with a response to a question that appears later in the questionnaire, so the interview is meant to be semi-structured. We therefore advise clinicians to make recordings of this part of the assessment so clinicians can fully focus on active listening.

As the clients respond to the questions, the clinician should invite them to elaborate by responding to follow-up questions such as: Can you expand on this? Can you tell me more? Can you give an example?

1. At what ages, respectively, were you diagnosed with cluttering and stuttering?
2. Did the diagnosis of cluttering bring about changes in your life? If so, please describe them.
3. Which disorder is more negatively stigmatized? Cluttering or stuttering?
4. Do you find that the symptoms of cluttering and stuttering influence each other? If so, how are they interrelated?
5. Which disorder affects you more, emotionally? Cluttering or stuttering?
6. What interferes more with your communication? Planning and formulating thoughts or fast and unclear speech?

7. Do you speak more than one language? If so, which languages do you speak? Which language is primary? Which language (primary or secondary) is affected more by cluttering and which by stuttering?
8. Which disorder is easier than the other to manage as a result of speech therapy? Cluttering or stuttering?
9. Do you believe that addressing cognitive and emotional aspects in cluttering therapy is as important as addressing them during stuttering therapy?
10. As a person with cluttering and stuttering, what progress do you expect to make, assuming you will consistently adhere to your speech therapy program?' ('Outstanding,' 'Good,' 'Fair,' or 'Poor'?)

Appendix H
Reading text for adult readers

Designed for adults, this reading material combines uplifting content with a comprehensive set of phonemes. Clinicians are encouraged to use this text consistently, comparing each client's speech performance to the performance of others.

The Secret of Happiness

Happiness has a magical attraction for humanity. Some seek bread, some seek wealth, and some seek fame, but all seek happiness. Most of us bend our efforts, more or less, to finding it and bringing it home. Unfortunately, only a few succeed. Most people do not understand where happiness can be found and naturally cannot obtain it. Some who succeed in finding happiness do not know how to nourish, develop, and preserve it. Consequently, it vanishes. It is easy to smile and be happy under pleasant conditions, but it takes a real optimist to see and find pleasure in life under adversity. That is the art of living. To know how to live is, after all, the best knowledge. A good way to find happiness is simply to be good, to be kind, and to develop in oneself an empathetic and optimistic view of things in the world, of its creatures, and fellow human beings. It is the pleasant feeling of kindness which makes a person happy. The more a person develops this feeling, the more such a person is sure of acquiring happiness.

Kindness is a general term. A noble character acquires happiness through the opportunity of making someone else happy. It is only that kind of kindness that will lead to happiness. When people develop a kindly opinion, a kindly thought, looking upon their environment through the light of kindness, they attract that power of electric magnetism – kindness. It forms an orbit of pleasantness and happiness around them. It develops in them a dynamo producing kindness with radiating power to influence their surroundings, thus creating a kind and happy atmosphere. To acquire the quality of kindness, which is a mental faculty, simply follow the method of physical acquirement – exercise. Athletes develop their muscles, their physical strength by practice. The same rule may apply to the mental qualities of kindness and happiness. People who practice kindness become kind and happy. There is no kind word or kind deed which does not have an effect, a return. Kindness is soft, flexible, springlike. Like a rubber ball, when one throws it at another, it bounces – it returns to oneself. Nothing wasted. Indeed, how badly our world needs kindness to make it happy! It is starved; it is as thirsty as the vegetation and the flowers in the dry desert anxiously awaiting a drop of moisture for the sustenance of life. What a pity! What a waste! How many beautiful flowers fade! How many worthy lives are wasted merely for the lack of a little dew, for a few drops of rain, or refreshing water, for a kind word, for a kind deed! A little water is not very much, but how much it does mean to the one who really needs it! It may mean the person's life. An act of kindness has a marvelous effect. It transforms the donor to the recipient. In consequence, it is not an expenditure, but it is an investment with an immediate return of high yield.

(Modified excerpt from *The Secret of Happiness* by David Miller, 1937)

Appendix I
Cluttering statement

My Speech Therapist
83–24 Cluttering Street
Disfluency Town

Cluttering statement

Place & Date: -   -

With this statement I declare that. . . . . (name), born
on. . . . . (birth date) and living in. . . . . (place) has been
diagnosed with cluttering.

Cluttering is a disorder of fluency that can lead to unintelligible or very
disfluent speech, sometimes in combination with language formulation problems. These symptoms occur at an uncontrollably fast rate of speech.

The problems that occur in cluttering increase with time pressure. If the
person with cluttering is able to focus and has enough time to formulate verbal and written speech tasks, this will lead to improved performance.

It is also advisable to provide special accommodations for students with
cluttering, as is done for students with dyslexia, e.g., headphones while taking reading tests, audio support while taking reading comprehension tests.
Some people with cluttering can be helped by using a feedback device during
oral testing.

Digitally signed in . . . . (Place). . . . . (Date). . . . .

The clinician

(Name). . . . .

Then send to parents.

Appendix J

Personal stories of people with cluttering and stuttering

The first three stories (Tanya, Charlene, and Baruti) are excerpted with permission from The *Stuttering Home Page*, Minnesota State University, Mankato https://web.mnsu.edu/comdis/kuster/stutter.html

From 'People with Cluttering and Stuttering Have Room for Success' by Tatyana Exum, Charlene Absalon, Baruti Smith and Isabella K. Reichel http://www.mnsu.edu/comdis/ica1/papers/exumc.html

Tanya

For many years, I was struggling with my communication problems as a student, as a teacher, and as a mother. A year ago, I searched the National Institute for Literacy Learning Disabilities listserv, where I started looking for an explanation of my speech difficulties which I had managed to 'cover up' for so long. I extensively described my experiences with my speech '. . . I could not pull out the word 'RESPECT' every time I needed it or why I tried to hurry up and finish my statements before I was . . . interrupted.' Why couldn't my frustrated teacher get any words out of me after the command to sit on my hands, while I was answering? Why could I not slow down with my speech, and just had to spit it out?' I got quite a few responses; however, the real answer came from an unexpected source – a speech pathologist who was evidently following our thread discussing issues relating to adults with learning disabilities, and who responded to one of my cries for help. She asked if I knew anything about cluttering and stuttering, and shared the ICA's website to assist me in my quest. A few days later, I hurried to inform her, 'According to all the materials I've read so far, I am a clutterer . . .' Very soon, we were constantly communicating on-line and on the phone. I was trying to catch up with the fireballs of her questions concerning the additional details I was sharing with her, which prompted the possibility of the coexisting issues, 'Does your sound come out with tension? Does your unclear speech make you frustrated? . . . Do you have an SLP in your town?' I was very surprised to find out that my hand movements were a secondary behavior which originally helped me to get through the word and that my feelings associated with my speech had an explanation. During our discussions, I kept revisiting my life experiences and reassessing the knowledge of myself. Our dialogue was unstoppable. Soon, she knew a lot more about me than people who surrounded me daily. My mind started filling up with the long-forgotten memories: my mom's effort to exclude the fill-ups in my speech; the lessons in piano and singing, when I had to use a metronome to slow me down; acting lessons, during which the sound production was addressed by putting marble balls in the mouth. Later, when I was exposed to the necessity of doing multiple presentations during my teaching career, I had to learn how to overcome blocks by playing them down as the intended pauses, or slapping my hand, by concentrating on the positive faces in the audience. I also had to learn how to overcome the wish to never open my mouth again after running sentences in an unknown direction and not looking smart. Delegating my speech controls to my students (they were my time keepers and reminded me to 'hit a space bar' when needed) happened to be one of my 'saving grace' tools. Through my discussions with [the speech pathologist referred to above], we discovered that my college course in Phonetics contained exercises also used in a speech pathology field. I started using these exercises again and found that by doing so, my speech started improving. There were two major components of our communication which helped tremendously in sorting things out: A very knowledgeable specialist, and a supportive ICA community with the availability of the resources on the website. Finding out my diagnosis and discussing my options made the whole experience invigorating. I felt such a sense of relief in knowing that what I had been experiencing was not my imagination; the problems were real; and they could be helped.

Charlene

Stuttering was never a big part of my life until I entered the world of adulthood and started to work in corporate America. Experiencing the stigma associated with stuttering was much harder than I had expected it to be. It began to set in every time I had a block and as a result I felt my personality change just to conform to the stuttering demon I had trapped inside. There were instances where my blocks would cause me to want to rip out my throat out of pure frustration. For years, I plastered on a fake smile to the world and hid the sadness in my eyes. Fluent speakers do not know that every pitied look or disgusted glance hurt ten times more than if I had been stabbed. Finally, after a few months at my second job, the anger gave me the determination to seek out the aid of a speech therapist. My first session with [my speech pathologist] was like letting the dam break free and letting the water run free. I remember crying, which I had always held inside, and telling her my story, and from then on, I began to feel healed. Every insulting look and smirk that I encountered once I got better slid off my back like water sliding off the waterproof feathers of a duck. My stuttering was minimized from a block every sentence to one block every two weeks. Once the issue of stuttering was resolved, another issue came to the forefront - cluttering. There were instances when my thoughts raced faster than my mouth could catch up. The competition usually resulted in a jumbled mass of words exiting my mouth, leaving both recipient and myself perplexed. Unlike stuttering, I was not ashamed about this problem. Instead, I shrugged it off as if a pesky bug, but it became an apparent problem when it became more frequent and when I would intend to say a word, but something completely different would come out. I always attributed this sort of mental dyslexia as normal, yet I had never heard another person jumble sentences into one verbal mass the way I did. I knew there was a problem, but denial is always easier to accept than the truth. It was a slow healing process, which I had to overcome. Between my second and third jobs, I was fluent for two years, with some minor relapses at times. I was hired for my third job as a fluent speaker, but the stress of the job and my personal life began to bear down on me and distracted me from thinking about the possibility of a relapse and practicing to maintain control of my speech. This led to a resumption of my stuttering and cluttering and brought on my current relapse with the same onslaught of emotions that attacked me in the past; however this time, I knew how to stop it from affecting me mentally. Now I began to work on my speech, practicing every other night, which helped decrease my blocks. To this day, the sadness has slowly crept out of my eyes again, but I am still working on regaining my natural smile rather than the mask. By practicing, I am able to bring myself to a higher foothold, a step closer to my freedom of speech. Despite my increase in blocks compared to when I had been down to about one every two weeks, I am 100 miles ahead of where I had been before I attended speech therapy.

Baruti

My name is Baruti Smith. In order to accomplish, one must have the attitude to do it. This is what I have learned over the years of overcoming my cluttering and stuttering. In my early years, especially in the stage in my life when I was in the 3rd grade, my speech problem first hit me. It was evident in the way my peers interacted with me. I began to make progress in this area when I made it my goal to be naturally accepted by other people without receiving sympathy. In the 7th grade I wasn't afraid to speak despite my speech issue. Let me add there is always frustration and an angry feeling that is a result of a speech impairment. I began to have success in my high school years, when I went to [a speech pathologist at a university clinic] for speech therapy and was diagnosed with cluttering and stuttering. First I thought it was a recipe for a lifetime of defeat and misunderstanding. I couldn't read normally either. I overcame my stuttering for good. I took it step by step; from phrases to simple sentences to paragraphs, etc. Since then I don't stutter at all. As a result of my speech therapy, my cluttering was mostly corrected as well. It cleared up so that it seemed like I had never stuttered or cluttered in the first place. I would make speeches in my speech therapist's classes; none of the students in the classroom realized that I had a cluttering or even a speech issue. After one and a half years of clear speech, after the completion of my therapy, my speech gradually got worse and I suffered a relapse of my cluttering. I'm not as bad as before, but at the same time I am not back to where I ought to be yet. So I can say I have tasted victory over cluttering for one and a half years, and then lost it. After a five-year break, I have now resumed speech therapy again. My present focus is on my cluttering. My philosophy is the better the mindset for success, the earlier one will get past one's troubles. I just want to encourage others to follow my lead in correcting speech issues. It is important to have ultimate confidence in yourself. As long as people work on their speech and maintain an attitude that they can overcome their cluttering and stuttering, they will be successful and accomplished!

Michael

This account is based on the experiences of a client of one of the authors. This client agreed to share his experiences with the use of an assumed name.

Michael, a 32-year-old successful accountant, sought treatment to address his unusual complaints of long duration. Although he had no speech or language disorders during regular communication, he encountered difficulties speaking when praying in a congregational setting and in front of small groups, including saying grace at festive meals with his family members. Michael stated that during such speaking situations, his speech rate escalated, resulting in fast and unclear speech, collapsing of syllables, lack of pauses and fear that people would not understand him. His frustration grew when his wife and his children wondered why no one in the family could understand what he was saying and offered ideas to make his speech clearer. As time went on, Michael developed anxiety when anticipating a call to recite blessings publicly in front of the congregation he attends. He silently prayed that his name would not be chosen. He exhibited some symptoms of hyperarousal typical for people with anxiety, such as heart palpitations, muscle tension and inadequate pauses to catch his breath during speaking. He went to a few speech pathologists, including some at a college speech clinic, and was invariably told that his condition was simply an abnormally fast speech rate at certain times, and he was assured that if only he would get used to speaking more slowly, all his problems would be resolved. Michael desperately tried to follow their advice, but without success. His anxiety, fear of embarrassment, low self-esteem, and negative beliefs about his speech gradually became unbearable, so he continued his search for help. Eventually he was seen by a clinician who explained Michael's speech symptoms as those characteristic of the fluency disorder of cluttering, which in his case only occurred during the public recitation of prayers that are viewed as automatic tasks where no programming and formulating ideas are required. Visibly relieved and excited, Michael embraced a new opportunity to try a treatment that required a commitment to change and adherence to a rigid schedule of exercises. Therapy addressed not only behavioral but also cognitive and affective aspects of cluttering. Bringing awareness of his symptoms gave him hope for recovery and motivation to practice. His speech intelligibility was addressed by working on grammatically appropriate breath group locations and duration which also contributed to the slowing down of his speech rate. The natural flow of his speech was facilitated by improving his speech rhythm and adequate intonational patterns. The clinician's strategies for reducing Michael's emotional arousal included discussing his negative beliefs, and implementing cognitive- behavioral and emotional intelligence concepts to address distorted thoughts about anticipated audiences' reactions. After eight sessions, Michael was happy to observe that his speech rate and intelligibility during prayers at home were completely normalized and that his cardiac and respiratory symptoms and muscle tension during congregational prayers almost disappeared.

Anjea Ray

Anjea Ray, a speech-language pathologist who was diagnosed with cluttering, is a co-author of an article that includes her story, which appears below.

Reichel, I. K., & Ray, A. (2008). The ICA adopts the cluttering orphan. *Perspectives on Fluency and Fluency Disorders, 18,* (2), 84–86.

Many individuals who stutter become SLPs to help others who suffer from the same condition. These SLPs enter the field armed with a much more personal understanding of the disorder that they wish to treat in others. But how often do SLPs enter the field unaware of their own speech difficulties and disfluencies? I have always been dubbed a 'fast talker,' and others have asked me to repeat myself or to slow down. My mother advised people that they would 'just have to learn to listen faster,' because she believed that my speaking patterns mirrored my outgoing, bubbly personality. As my family was habituated to my speech, they never thought anything errant about it. I never did, either, until I began my graduate studies in communication disorders to become an SLP.I consistently received positive feedback for my clinical work, but every one of my supervisors, in addition to the other faculty members, commented on my rate of speech. I thought I was speaking more slowly after these persistent reminders, but apparently my perception and that of my supervisors, fellow student clinicians, and clients did not match. It wasn't until my fluency professor told me that I needed to 'stop this cluttering business to truly succeed as a speech-language pathologist' that I realized it was a real problem. He had labeled my speech and I didn't know what that label meant or its potential implications for my future career path. After some research, a phone call to Dr. Kenneth St. Louis, some self-analysis, and more consultations with my fluency professor and supervisors, I acknowledged and accepted that I was indeed a clutterer. I became extremely self-conscious as

I began to notice more and more disfluencies in my speech—repetition of words/syllables, omission of sounds within words, abrupt/abnormal pauses, poor verbal organization, and 'rushes' of speech (an incoherent, poorly articulated gibberish that only my closest friends can understand within a known context) formed with incomplete sentences without transitions. As my awareness increased, so did my stress from clinical rotations, my ongoing frustration with my inability to break the speech patterns, and my mounting fear of being ineffective as a SLP working with cognitively and linguistically impaired populations and their families. The awareness of how my cluttered speech would affect my success as a clinician spurred my interest in the disorder—in particular, its management. My professor advised me to take a behavioral approach—to think about moving slowly, rather than talking slowly, and to feel each sound as I produced it. That has probably helped the most, coupled with Dr. St. Louis' advice about practicing reading aloud (and in particular, poetry) while recording myself and analyzing my own speech to better understand the patterns specific to my speech. I try to organize my thoughts in my head before I express them, in an effort to keep the ideas linear, clear, and concise; this skill is critical for SLPs in general, but arguably more so for me as I work with the elderly in a nursing home.

Appendix K
Reading passages

My grandfather

You wish to know all about my grandfather. Well, he is nearly 93 years old, yet he still thinks as swiftly as ever. He dresses himself in an ancient, black frock coat, usually minus several buttons. A long, flowing beard clings to his chin, giving those who observe him a pronounced feeling of the utmost respect. When he speaks his voice is just a bit cracked and quivers a trifle. Twice each day he plays skillfully and with zest upon a small organ. Except in the winter when the snow or ice prevents, he slowly takes a short walk in the open air each day. We have often urged him to walk more and smoke less but he always answers, 'Banana oil!' Grandfather likes to be modern in his language.

The rainbow

When the sunlight strikes raindrops in the air, they act like a prism and form a rainbow. A rainbow is the division of white light into many beautiful colors. These take the shape of a large, round arch, with its path high above and its two ends apparently beyond the horizon. There is, according to legend, a boiling pot of gold at one end. People look, but no one ever finds it. When a man looks for something beyond his reach, his friends say he is looking for the pot of gold at the end of the rainbow.

Limpy

Limpy is a fuzzy, yellow, baby duck. He belongs to a fisherman. The fisherman lives in a little house by the bay. Every morning children go swimming in the bay. About 10:00, Limpy waddles out to the road to wait for the children. When he hears them coming he begins a loud, excited quacking. The children always bring bread or corn for Limpy. He will nip at their fingers or peck at their bare toes until he is fed. Limpy never follows the children down to the shore. He likes to swim in his own little pond. It is much safer.

Appendix L
Speech Situation Checklist for cluttering

(Adapted from Brutten & Shoemaker, 1981)

Goal

With the help of the Speech Situation Checklist, the client will become aware of the level of complexity of diverse speaking situations. If clients start to practice new skills in their daily life situations, these levels of complexity have to be taken into account. The list developed for people with stuttering is adjusted for people with cluttering. In the column of disturbed speech, attention is given to poor intelligibility, fast or irregular rate, pauses in the linguistically inappropriate places, and the production of an excessive number of normal disfluencies. Normative data for the questionnaire are only available for stuttering (Behavior Assessment Battery, 2007).

Procedure

Ask the client to complete the table. Provide the following instructions:

1 First fill in the right column, 'disturbed speech.'
2 Temporarily cover over the right column so you cannot see it.
3 Fill in the left column, 'emotional response,' a day later.
4 Compare the scores.

Tip: Compute a separate mean score each time. For example: talking on the phone is dependent on the topic or the person. Compute a mean score.

Scores

1 not at all
2 a little bit
3 pretty much
4 a lot
5 very much

Speech Situation Checklist (adapted from Brutten & Shoemaker, 1981)

Name:
Date:

Situation	Emotional response	Disturbed speech
1 having a telephone conversation		
2 talking to a stranger		
3 giving one's own name or introducing oneself		
4 talking to a small child		
5 producing a word or sentence that gave difficulties earlier		
6 ordering in a restaurant		
7 talking to an animal		
8 asking to be forwarded on the phone to a certain person		
9 having a conversation with a good friend		
10 having an argument with parents or a partner		
11 talking to a sales person		
12 participating in a group conversation		
13 receiving criticism		
14 meeting someone for the first time		
15 talking after being criticized		
16 talking after being misunderstood		
17 saying hello		
18 reading an unknown text out loud		
19 responding to a certain question		
20 being interviewed for a job		
21 asking for information		
22 trying to convince other people		
23 talking through skype or facetime		
24 giving instructions		
25 talking after drinking some alcohol		

Situation	Emotional response	Disturbed speech
26 talking with a hairstylist		
27 trying to impress someone		
28 speaking when depressed		
29 talking to teachers or authorities		
30 making an appointment		
31 asking a question in a classroom or office meeting		
32 answering questions about one's speech		
33 repeating an answer		
34 talking when at home		
35 introducing a friend to a friend		
36 giving one's personal data (name, address, etc.)		
37 talking when tired		
38 buying a ticket to a certain destination		
39 presenting in front of a big group		
40 presenting in front of a small group		
41 presenting without preparation		
42 being rushed during speech		
43 explaining important issues to friends		
44 talking in a bar		
45 discussing a sporting event		
46 talking while playing a computer game		
47 telling a joke		

References

Alahari, U. (2017). Supporting socio-emotional competence and psychological well-being of school psychologists through mindfulness practice. *Contemporary School Psychology*, *21*, 369–379. doi: 10.1007/s40688-017-0154-x

Al-Khaledi, M., Lincoln, M., McCabe, P., Packman, A., & Alshatti, T. (2009). The attitudes, knowledge and beliefs of Arab parents in Kuwait about stuttering. *Folia Phoniatrica et Logopaedica*, *34*(1), 44–59.

Allington, R.L., McCuiston, K., & Billen, M. (2015). What research says about text complexity and learning to read. *The reading teacher*, *68*(7), 491–501. https://doi.org/10.1002/trtr.1280

Alm, P. (2008, July). *Fluency disorders: A discussion of possible causes and mechanisms, from a neuroscience perspective*. Contribution to Oxford Dysfluency Congress, Oxford.

Alm, P. (2011). Cluttering: A neurological perspective. In D. Ward & K. Scaler Scott (eds.), *Cluttering: A handbook of research, intervention and education* (pp. 3–28). Psychology Press.

Andrade, C.R. de & Oliveira Martins, V. de (2010). Speech fluency variation in elderly. *Pró-Fono Revista de Atualização Científica*, *22*(1), 13–18.

Apple, W., Streeter, L.A., & Krauss, R.M. (1979). Effects of pitch and speech rate on personal attributions. *Journal of Personality and Social Psychology*, *37*(5), 715–727. https://doi.org/10.1037/0022-3514.37.5.715

Arenas (2014). Speech Monitor [DAF/FAF software]. www.speechmonitor.org

Autisme Spectrum Centrum (2022). https://www.autismespectrumcentrum.nl/wat-is-autisme

Bakker, K. (1996). Cluttering: Current scientific status and emerging research and clinical needs. *Journal of Fluency Disorders*, *21*(3–4), 359–366.

Bakker, K., Myers, F.L., Raphael, L.J., & St. Louis, K.O. (2011). A preliminary comparison of speech rate, self-evaluation, and disfluency of people who speak exceptionally fast, clutter, or speak normally. In D. Ward & K. Scaler Scott (eds.), *Cluttering: A handbook of research, intervention and education* (pp. 45–65). Psychology Press.

Bakker, K., Raphael, L.J., Myers, F.L., & St. Louis, K.O. (2000). *Acoustic and perceptual-phonetic analyses of cluttered and noncluttered speech*. Paper presented at the Annual Convention of the American Speech-Language-Hearing Association, Washington, D.C.

Bakker, K., St. Louis, K.O., Myers, F., & Raphael, L. (2005). *A freeware software tool for determining aspects of cluttering severity*. Paper presented at the Annual Convention of the American Speech-Language-Hearing Association, San Diego, CA.

Bangert, K.J., Scaler Scott, K., Adams, C., Kisenwether, J.S., Giuffre, L., Reed, J., John Thurman, A., Abbeduto, L., & Klusek, J. (2022). Cluttering in the Speech of Males with Fragile X Syndrome, *Journal of Speech, Language, and Hearing Research*, 65(3), 954–969.

Bargh, J.A. (1994). The Four Horsemen of automaticity: Awareness, efficiency, intention, and control in social cognition. In R.S. Wyer Jr., & T.K. Srull (eds.), *Handbook of social cognition* (2nd ed.), (pp. 1–40). Erlbaum.

Barnes, E., Roberts, J., Long, S., Martin, G.E., Berni, M.C., Mandulak, K.C., & Sideris, J. (2009). Phonological accuracy and intelligibility in connected speech of boys with fragile X syndrome or Down syndrome. *Journal of Speech, Language, and Hearing Research*, 52(4), 1048–1061.

Bar-On, R. (2000). Emotional and social intelligence: Insights from the emotional quotient inventory. In R. Bar-On & J.D.A. Parker (eds.), *The handbook of emotional intelligence* (pp. 363–388). Jossey-Bass.

Baumgartner, J. (1999). Acquired psychogenic stuttering. In R.F. Curlee (ed.), *Stuttering and related disorders of stuttering and related disorders of fluency* (pp. 269–288). Thieme.

Becker, K.P., & Grundmann, K. (1970). Investigation on incidence and symptomatology of cluttering. *Folia Phoniatrica et Logopaedica*, 22(4–5), 261–271.

Bennett Lanouette, E. (2011). Intervention strategies for cluttering disorders. In D. Ward & K. Scaler Scott (eds.), *Cluttering: A handbook of research, intervention and education* (pp. 175–197). Psychology Press.

Bennett, E.M. (2006). *Working with people who stutter: A lifespan approach*. Pearson Merrill Prentice-Hall.

Bezemer, B.W., Bouwen, J., & Winkelman, C. (2010). *Stotteren: Van theorie naar therapie*. Coutinho.

Blake, D.T., Heiser, M.A., Caywood, M., & Merzenich, M.M. (2006). Experience-dependent adult cortical plasticity requires cognitive association between sensation and reward. *Neuron*, 52(2), 371–381.

Block, S. (2004). The evidence base for the treatment of stuttering. In S. Reilly, J. Douglas & J. Oates (eds.), *Evidence based practice in speech pathology* (pp. 330–352). Whurr.

Blokker, M., Vos, S., & Wingerden, K. van (2010). *Normale niet-vloeiendheden in adolescenten met dyslexie* [bachelor thesis]. Hogeschool Utrecht.

Boersma, P., & Weenink, D. (2022). *Praat: Doing phonetics by computer*. [Software]. www.praat.org

Bóna, J., & Kohári, A. (2021). Rate vs. rhythm characteristics of cluttering with data from a 'syllable-timed' language. *Journal of Fluency Disorders*, 67, 105801. https://doi.org/10.1016/j.jfludis.2020.105801

Bóna, J. (2019). Clustering of disfluencies in typical, fast and cluttered speech. *Clinical Linguistics & Phonetics*, 33(5), 393–405.

Bóna, J. (2021). Self-initiated error-repairs in cluttering. *Clinical Linguistics & Phonetics*, 35(5), 405–418. https://doi.org/10.1080/02699206.2020.1787521

Bothe, A.K. (2008). Identification of children's stuttered and nonstuttered speech by highly experienced judges: Binary judgments and comparisons with disfluency-types definitions. *Journal of Speech, Language, and Hearing Research*, 51(4), 867–878.

Boyle, M.P. (2011). Mindfulness training in stuttering therapy: A tutorial for speech-language pathologists. *Folia Phoniatrica et Logopaedica*, 36(2), 122–129.

Bradlow, A. R. (2019). Speaking Rate, Information Density, and Information Rate in First-Language and Second-Language Speech. In *INTERSPEECH* (pp. 3559–3563).

Bray, M. (2003). *Monica Bray's survey looks at dysfluency in Down's syndrome and at the success or otherwise of different treatment approaches*. http://www.stammering.org/downs_survey.html

Bretherton-Furness, J., & Ward, D. (2012). Lexical access, story re-telling and sequencing skills in adults who clutter and those who do not. *Folia Phoniatrica et Logopaedica, 37*(4), 214–224.

Britto Pereira, M.M. de, Rossi, J.P., & Van Borsel, J. (2008). Public awareness and knowledge of stuttering in Rio de Janeiro. *Journal of Fluency Disorders, 33*(1), 24–31.

Brutten, G., & Janssen, P. (1981). *A normative and factor analysis study of the responses of Dutch and American stutterers to the Speech Situation Checklist.* Proceedings 18th. Congress International Association of Logopedics and Phoniatrists, USA 80, 281–286.

Brutten, G. & Shoemaker, D. (1981). Speech Situation Checklist. In The Southern Illinois Checklist. Carbondale, IL: Southern Illinois University.

Brutten, G. (1979). Vragenlijst spreeksituaties. In P. Janssen (ed.), *Gedragstherapie bij stotteren.* Bohn Stafleu van Loghum.

Brutten, G. (1981). The Speech Situation Checklist: Comments on its use as a measure of severity. *Logopedie en Foniatrie, 52,* 472–476.

Burger, E., Wetering, M. van & Weerdenburg, M. van (eds.) (2012). *Kinderen met specifieke taalstoornissen: (Be)handelen en begeleiden in zorg en onderwijs.* Acco.

Burken, P. van, Boer, T.C. de & Browne, G. (2017). *Mindfulness en fysiotherapie.* Bohn Stafleu van Loghum.

Burt, L., Holm, A., & Dodd, B. (1999). Phonological awareness skills of 4-year-old British children: An assessment and developmental data. *International Journal of Language & Communication Disorders, 34*(3), 311–335. https://doi.org/10.1080/136828299247432

Chon, H, Sawyer, J, & Ambrose, N.G. Differences of articulation rate and utterance length in fluent and disfluent utterances of preschool children who stutter. *J Commun Disord.* 2012; 45(6):455–67.

Colombat de L'Isère, M. (1849). Les maladies de la voix et les vices de la parole. *Journal de Réadaptation Médicale, 23*(1–2), 54–60.

Conture, E.D., & Curlee, R.F. (eds.) (2007). *Stuttering and related disorders of fluency* (3rd ed.). Thieme.

Coppens-Hofman, M.C., Terband, H.R., Maassen, B.A.M., Schrojenstein Lantman-de Valk, H.M.J., Zaalen-op 't Hof, Y. van & Snik, A.F.M. (2013). Dysfluencies in the speech of adults with intellectual disabilities and reported speech difficulties. *Journal of Communication Disorders, 46*(5–6), 484–494.

Cosyns, M., Meulemans, M., Vermeulen, E., Busschots, L., Corthals, P., & Van Borsel, J. (2018). Measuring articulation rate: A comparison of two methods. *Journal of Speech, Language, and Hearing Research,* 61(11), 2772–2778.

Cosyns, M., Mortier, G., Janssens, S., Bogaert, F., D'Hondt, S., & Van Borsel, J. (2012). Articulation in schoolchildren and adults with neurofibromatosis type 1. *Journal of Communication Disorders, 45*(2), 111–120. https://doi.org/10.1016/j.jcomdis.2011.11.002

Cosyns, M., Zaalen-op 't Hof, Y. van, Mortier, G., Janssens, S., Amez, A., Van Damme, J., & Van Borsel, J. (2013). Disfluency: It is not always stuttering. *Clinical Genetics, 85*(3), 298–299.

Dalton, P., & Hardcastle, W. (1993). *Disorders of fluency and their effects on communication* (2nd ed.). Whurr.

Daly, D.A., & Burnett, M.L. (1996). Cluttering: Assessment, treatment planning, and case study illustration. *Journal of Fluency Disorders, 21*(3–4), 239–248.

Daly, D.A., & Burnett, M.L. (1999). Cluttering: Traditional views and new perspectives. In R.F. Curlee (eds.), *Stuttering and disorders of fluency* (2nd ed.). (pp. 222–254). Thieme.

Daly, D.A., & Cantrell, R.P. (2006). *Cluttering characteristics identified as diagnostically significant by 60 fluency experts.* Paper presented at the Second World Congress on Fluency Disorders van de International Fluency Association, Dublin.

Daly, D.A. (1986). The clutterer. In K.O. St. Louis (eds.), *The atypical stutterer: Principles and practice of rehabilitation* (pp. 155–192). Academic Press.

Daly, D.A. (1992). Helping the clutterer: Therapy considerations. In F. Myers & K.O. St. Louis (eds.). *Cluttering: A clinical perspective* (pp. 107–124). FAR Communications.

Daly, D.A. (1993). Cluttering: Another fluency syndrome. In: R. Curlee (ed.), *Stuttering and related disorders of fluency*. Thieme Medical Publishers, Inc.

Daly, D.A. (1996). *The source for stuttering and cluttering*. LinguiSystems.

Daly, D.A. (2008). *Cluttering: A language-based syndrome*. [Audio]. Clinical Connection.

Damsté, P.H. (1984). *Stotteren: Onwillekeurig of willekeurig gedrag?* (3rd ed.). Bohn, Scheltema & Holkema.

Damsté, P.H. (1990). *Stotteren: Onwillekeurig of willekeurig gedrag?* (4th ed.). Bohn, Scheltema & Holkema.

Dannenbauer, F.M. (1999). Grammatik. In G. Baumgartner & J. Fussenich (eds.), *Sprachtherapie mit Kindern* (pp. 105–161). E. Reinhardt.

De Nil, L.F., Jokel, R., & Rochon, E. (2007). Etiology, symptomatology, and treatment of neurogenic stuttering. In E.G. Conture & R.F. Curlee (eds.), *Stuttering and related disorders of fluency* (3rd ed.). (pp. 326–343). Thieme.

De Nil, L.F., Sasisekaran, J., Lieshout, P.H.H.M. van & Sandor, P. (2005). Speech disfluencies in individuals with Tourette syndrome. *Journal of Psychosomatic Research*, 58(1), 97–102.

De Puzzelmaker (2021). Zoek de verschillen. https://depuzzelmaker.nl/zoek-de-verschillen-2/

Deckers, S.R., Zaalen, Y. van & Reichel, I. (2015). *Speech and fluency development in children with Down syndrome*. Poster presented at the Touro College, New York.

Deckers, S.R., Zaalen, Y. van, Balkom, H. van & Verhoeven, L. (2019). Predictors of receptive and expressive vocabulary development in children with Down syndrome. *International Journal of Speech-Language Pathology*, 21(1), 10–22.

deHirsch, K. (1961). Studies in tachyphemia: Diagnosis of developmental language disorders. *Logos*, 4(1), 3–9.

deHirsch, K. (1970). Stuttering and cluttering: Developmental aspects of dysrhythmic speech. *Folia Phoniatrica et Logopaedica*, 22(4), 311–324.

Devenny, D., & Silverman, W. (1990). Speech dysfluency and manual specialization in Down's syndrome. *Journal of Mental Deficiency Research*, 34(3), 253–260.

Diedrich, W.M. (1984). Cluttering: Its diagnosis. In: H. Winitz (eds.), *Treating articulation disorders: For clinicians by clinicians* (pp. 307–323). University Park Press.

Dinger, T., Smit, M., & Winkelman, C. (2008). *Expressiever en gemakkelijker spreken*. Coutinho.

Dodd, B., & Thompson, L. (2001). Speech disorder in children with Down's syndrome. *Journal of Intellectual Disability Research*, 45(4), 308–316. https://doi.org/10.1046/j.1365-2788.2001.00327

Dodd, B. (1995). *The differential diagnosis and treatment of children with speech disorders* (Ser. Studies in disorders of communication). Whurr.

Drayna, D. (2011). Possible genetic factors in cluttering. In D. Ward & K. Scaler Scott (eds.), *Cluttering: A handbook of research, intervention and education* (pp. 29–33). Psychology Press.

Dyslexia Fund Foundation (n.d.). *What is dyslexia?* https://dyslexie.nl/wat-is-dyslexie

Eggers, K., & Van Eerdenbrugh, S. (2018). Speech disfluencies in children with Down Syndrome. *Journal of Communication Disorders*, 71, 72–84. https://doi.org/10.1016/j.jcomdis.2017.11.001

Eggers, K. (2010, August). *What is normal dysfluency and why measure it?* Paper presented at the 28th World Congress of the International Association of Logopedics and Phoniatrics, Athene.

Eisenson, J. (1986). Dysfluency disorders: Cluttering and stuttering. In A. Goldstein, L. Krasner & S. Garfield (eds.), *Language and speech disorders in children* (pp. 57–75). Pergamon.

Eldridge, K.A. (2007). *Phonological complexity and speech disfluency in young children* [Doctoral dissertation, University of Pittsburgh], Dietrich School of Communication Science and Disorders.

Engelhardt, P.E., Corley, M., Nigg, J.T., & Ferreira, F. (2010). The role of inhibition in the production of disfluencies. *Memory & Cognition*, 38(5), 617–628. https://doi.org/10.3758/MC.38.5.617

Exum, T., Absalon, C., Smith, B., & Reichel, I.K. (2010). *People with cluttering and stuttering have room for success.* Paper presented at the International Cluttering Online Conference, Minnesota State University, Mankato, MN. Opgevraagd van http://www.mnsu.edu/comdis/ica1/papers/exumc.html

Ezell, J., Hogan, A., Fairchild, A., Hills, K., Klusek, J., Abbeduto, L., & Roberts, J. (2019). Prevalence and predictors of anxiety disorders in adolescent and adult males with autism spectrum disorder and fragile X syndrome. *Journal of Autism and Developmental Disorders*, 49(3), 1131–1141. https://doi.org/10.1007/s10803-018-3804-6

Filatova, Y.O. (2005). [*Cluttering*]. Prometey.

Florenskaya, J.A. (1934). A question about functional speech disorders: Paraphasia and tachylalia. *Contemporary Psychoneurology, 4*.

Freund, H. (1952). Studies in the interrelationship between stuttering and cluttering. *Folia Phoniatrica et Logopaedica*, 4(3), 146–168.

Freund, H. (1966). *Psychopathology and the problems of stuttering.* Charles C. Thomas.

Freund, H. (1970). Observations on tachylalia. *Folia Phoniatrica et Logopaedica*, 22(4), 280–288.

Friedmann, N., Biran, M., & Dotan, D. (2013). Lexical retrieval and its breakdown in aphasia and developmental language impairment. In C. Boeckx & K.K. Grohmann (eds.), *The Cambridge handbook of biolinguistics* (pp. 350–374). Cambridge University Press.

Froeschels, E. (1946). Cluttering. *Journal of Speech Disorders*, 11(1), 31–33.

Garnett, E.O., Adams, C.F., Montgomery, A.A., St. Louis, K.O., & Ouden, D.B. den (2012). *Phonological encoding in cluttering.* Poster presented at the 7th World Congress on Fluency Disorders of the International Fluency Association, Tours.

Georgieva, D. (2004). Professional awareness of cluttering: A comparative study (Part Two). In H.-G. Bosshardt, J.S. Yaruss & H.F. Peters (eds.), *Fluency disorders: Theory, research, treatment, and self-help: Proceedings of the Fourth World Congress on Fluency Disorders* (pp. 630–634). International Fluency Association.

Georgieva, D. (2010). Understanding cluttering: Eastern European traditions vs. Western European and North American traditions. In K. Bakker, L. Raphael & F. Myers (eds.), *Proceedings of the First International Conference on Cluttering* (pp. 230–243). International Cluttering Association.

Gillberg, J. (1992). Subgroups in autism: Are there behavioural phenotypes typical of underlying medical conditions? *Journal of Intellectual Disability Research*, 36(3), 201–214.

Green, T. (1999). The cluttering problem: A short review and a critical comment. *Logopedics Phoniatrics Vocology*, 24(4), 145–153.

Gutzmann, H. (1893). *Vorlesungen über die Störungen der Sprache und ihre Heilung.* Kornfeld.

Hagerman, R.J., Berry-Kravis, E., Hazlett, H.C., Bailey, D.B., Moine, H., Kooy, R.F., Tassone, F., Gantois, I., Sonenberg, N., Mandel, J.L., & Hagerman, P.J. (2017). Fragile X syndrome. *Nature Reviews. Disease Primers*, 3(17065). https://doi.org/10.1038/nrdp.2017.65

Hall, K.D., Amir, O., & Yairi, E. (1999). A longitudinal investigation of speaking rate in preschool children who stutter. *Journal of Speech, Language, and Hearing Research*, 42(6), 1367–1377.

Hartinger, M., & Mooshammer, C. (2008). Articulatory variability in cluttering. *Folia Phoniatrica et Logopaedica, 60*(2), 64–72.

Hartingsveldt, M. van, Cup, E., & Corstens-Mignot, M. (2010). *Korte Observatie Ergotherapie Kleuters (KOEK)*. Ergoboek.

Heeswijk, E. van (2011). *Influence of narrative task on linguistic fluency in syntactic cluttering* [Master's thesis]. Universiteit Utrecht.

Hernandez, A. E. (2009). Language switching in the bilingual brain: What's next? *Brain and Language, 109(2–3), 133–140.*

Hoorn, J.F. van, Maathuis, C.G., Peters, L.H., & Hadders-Algra, M.I.J.N.A. (2010). Handwriting, visuomotor integration, and neurological condition at school age. *Developmental Medicine & Child Neurology, 52*(10), 941–947.

Howell, P., & Au-Yeung, J. (2002). The EXPLAN theory of fluency control and the diagnosis of stuttering. In E. Fava (eds.), *Clinical linguistics: Theory and applications in speech pathology and therapy* (pp. 75–94). John Benjamins.

Howell, P., & Davis, S. (2011). The epidemiology of cluttering with stuttering. In D. Ward & K. Scaler Scott (eds.), *Cluttering: A handbook of research, intervention and education* (pp. 69–89). Psychology Press.

Howell, P. (2004). Assessment of some contemporary theories of stuttering that apply to spontaneous speech. *Contemporary Issues in Communication Science and Disorders, 31, 122–139.*

Hunt, J. (1861). *Stammering and stuttering: Their nature and treatment.* Longmans, Green, Longman and Roberts.

Hunter, J., Rivero-Arias, O., Angelov, A., Kim, E., Fotheringham, I., & Leal, J. (2014). Epidemiology of fragile X syndrome: A systematic review and meta-analysis. *American Journal of Medical Genetics, 164*(7), 1648–1658.

Jang, Y.E., & Shin, M.S. (2021). Characteristics of reading fluency and speech fluency in school-age ADHD children and stuttering children. *Journal of Speech, Language and Hearing Disorders, 30*(4), 95–103. https://doi.org/10.15724/jslhd.2021.30.4.095

Janssen, P. (1985). *Gedragstherapie bij stotteren.* Bohn, Scheltema & Holkema.

Jerome, L. (2003). Some observations on the phenomenology of thought disorder: A neglected sign in attention-deficit hyperactivity disorder. *Journal of the Canadian Academy of Child and Adolescent Psychiatry, 12*(3), 92–93.

Johnson, M.K., & Hasher, L. (1987). Human learning and memory. In M.R. Rosenzweig & L.W. Porter (eds.), *Annual review of psychology* (pp. 631–668). Annual Reviews.

Juste, F., Rondon, S., & Sassi, F.C. (2012). Acoustic analyses of diadochokinesis in fluent and stuttering children. *Clinics, 67*(5), 409–414.

Kabat-Zinn, J. (1994). *Wherever you go, there you are: Mindfulness meditation in everyday life.* Hyperion.

Kabat-Zinn, J. (2000). Indra's net at work: The mainstreaming of Dharma practice in society. In G. Watson, S. Batchelor & G. Claxton (eds.), *The psychology of awakening: Buddhism, science, and our day-to-day lives* (pp. 225–249). Samuel Weiser.

Kaczynska, J., & Janik, P. (2021). Blocking tics in Gilles de la Tourette syndrome. *Frontiers in Neurology, 12, 686785.* https://doi.org/10.3389/fneur.2021.686785

Kahneman, D., & Treisman, A. (1984). Changing views of attention and automaticity. In R. Parasuraman, D.R. Davies & J. Beatty (eds.), *Varieties of attention* (pp. 29–61). Academic Press.

Kaipa, R., Jones, R.D., & Robb, M.P. (2016). Are individuals with Parkinson's disease capable of speech-motor learning? A preliminary evaluation. *Parkinsonism & Related Disorders, 28, 141–145.* https://doi.org/10.1016/j.parkreldis.2016.05.001

Kallinen, K., & Ravaja, N. (2004). Emotion-related effects of speech rate and rising vs. falling background music melody during audio news: The moderating influence of personality. *Personality and Individual Differences, 37*(2), 275–288. https://doi.org/10.1016/j.paid.2003.09.002

Karlsdottir, R., & Stefansson, T. (2002). Problems in developing functional handwriting. *Perceptual and Motor Skills, 94*(2), 623–662.

Kelly, E.M., & Conture, G. (1992). Speaking rates, response time latencies, and interrupting behaviors of young stutterers, nonstutterers, and their mothers. *Journal of Speech, Language, and Hearing Research, 35*(6), 1256–1267.

Kempen, G., & Hoenkamp, E. (1987). An incremental procedural grammar for sentence formulation. *Cognitive Science, 11*(2), 201–258.

Kent, R.D. (1984). Stammering as a temporal programming disorder. In R.F. Curlee & W. Perkins (eds.), *Nature and treatment of stammering: New directions* (pp. 283–301). College Hill Press.

Kinoshita, S., & Verdonschot, R.G. (2021). Phonological encoding is free from orthographic influence: Evidence from a picture variant of the phonological Stroop task. *Psychological Research, 85*(3), 1340–1347. https://doi.org/10.1007/s00426-020-01315-2

Knock, T.R., Ballard, K.J., Robin, D.A., & Schmidt, R.A. (2000). Influence of order of stimulus presentation on speech motor learning: A principled approach to treatment for apraxia of speech. *Aphasiology, 14*(5–6), 653–668. https://doi.org/10.1080/026870300401379

Kochergina, V.S. (1969). Bradylalia, tachylalia, dysfluency. In S.S. Lyapidevsky (ed.), *Speech impairment in children and adolescents* (pp. 213–226). Prosveshtenie.

Krivokapić, J., Styler, W., & Parrell, B. (2020). Pause postures: the relationship between articulation and cognitive processes during pauses. *Journal of Phonetics, 79,* 100953. https://doi.org/10.1016/j.wocn.2019.100953

Kumin, L., & Adams, J. (2000). Developmental apraxia of speech and intelligibility in children with Down syndrome. *Down Syndrome Quarterly, 5*(3), 1–7.

Kumin, L. (2006). *Early communication skills for children with Down syndrome: A guide for parents and professionals* (Ser. Topics in Down syndrome). Woodbine House.

Kussmaul, A. (1877). Diseases of the nervous system and disturbances of speech. In H. von Ziemssen (ed.), *Cyclopedia of the practice of medicine* (Chapter 27). William Wood.

Langevin, M., & Boberg, E. (1996). Results of intensive stuttering therapy with adults who clutter and stutter. *Journal of Fluency Disorders, 21*(3–4), 315–328.

Langová, J., & Morávek, M. (1964). Some results of experimental examinations among stutterers and clutterers. *Folia Phoniatrica et Logopaedica, 16,* 290–296.

Langová, J., & Morávek, M. (1970). Some problems of cluttering. *Folia Phoniatrica et Logopaedica, 22*(4), 325–326.

Lebrun, Y. (1996). Cluttering after brain damage. *Journal of Fluency Disorders, 21,* 289–296.

Levelt, W.J.M. (1983). Monitoring and self-repair in speech. *Cognition, 14*(1), 41–104.

Levelt, W.J.M. (1989). *Speaking: From intention to articulation.* MIT Press.

Levelt, W.J.M. (1992). Accessing words in speech production: Stages, processes and representations. *Cognition, 42*(1–3), 1–22.

Levelt, W.J.M. (1993). Lexical selection, or how to bridge the major rift in language processing. In F. Beckmann, G. Heyer & W. de Gruyter (eds.), *Theorie und Praxis des Lexikons* (pp. 164–172). Walter De Gruyter.

Light, J. (1997). "Communication is the essence of human life": Reflections on communicative competence. *Augmentative and Alternative Communication, 13*(2), 61–70.

Logan, G.D., & Cowan, W.B. (1984). On the ability to inhibit thought and action: A theory of an act of control. *Psychological Review, 91*(3), 295–327.

Logan, K.J., & LaSalle, L.R. (1999). Grammatical characteristics of children's conversational utterances that contain disfluency clusters. *Journal of Speech, Language, and Hearing Research, 42*(1), 80–91.

Longcamp, M., Hlushchuk, Y., & Hari, R. (2011). What differs in visual recognition of handwritten vs. printed letters? An fMRi study. *Human Brain Mapping, 32*(8), 1250–1259.

Luchsinger, R., & Arnold, G.E. (1965). Cluttering: Tachyphemia. In R. Luchsinger & G.E. Arnold (eds.), *Voice-Speech-Language: Clinical communicology: Its physiology and pathology* (pp. 598–618). Wadsworth.

Luchsinger, R., & Arnold, G.E. (1970). *Handbuch der Stimm- und Sprachheilkunde.* Springer.

Luchsinger, R., & Landholt, H. (1955). Über das Poltern, das sogenannte 'Stottern mit Polterkomponente' und deren Beziehung zu den Aphasien [About cluttering, the so-called 'stutter with cluttering component' and its relations to aphasia]. *Folia Phoniatrica et Logopaedica, 7*(1), 12–43.

Luchsinger, R. (1951). Remarks to the history of phoniatrics in the eighteenth century, *Folia Phoniatrica et Logopaedica, 3,* 178–183.

Luchsinger, R. (1963). *Poltern.* Manhold.

Maassen, B., & Bastiaanse, R. (1996). Het Taal- en Spraakproductiemodel van Levelt. *Stem-, Spraak- en Taalpathologie, 5*(3), 127–133.

Maeland, A.F. (1992). Handwriting and perceptual-motor skills in clumsy, dysgraphic, and 'normal' children. *Perceptual and Motor Skills, 75*(3), 1207–1217. https://doi.org/10.2466/pms.1992.75.3f.12

Marklund, U., Marklund, E., Lacerda, F., & Schwarz, I. (2015). Pause and utterance duration in child-directed speech in relation to child vocabulary size. *Journal of Child Language, 42*(5), 1158–1171. https://doi.org/10.1017/S0305000914000609

Marquardt, C., Meyer, M.D., Schneider, M., & Hilgemann, R. (2016). Learning handwriting at school: A teachers' survey on actual problems and future options. *Trends in Neuroscience and Education, 5*(3), 82–89. https://doi.org/10.1016/j.tine.2016.07.001

Martínez-Sánchez, F., Meilán, J.J.G., Carro, J., Íñiguez, C.G., Millian-Morell, L., Pujante Valverde, I.M., López-Alburquerque, T., & López, D.E. (2016). Speech rate in Parkinson's disease: A controlled study. *Neurología (English Edition), 31*(7), 466–472.

Mayer, J.D., Salovey, P., & Caruso, D.R. (2000). Models of emotional intelligence. In R.J. Sternberg (eds.), *Handbook of intelligence* (pp. 396–420). Cambridge University Press.

Melbourne Academic Mindfulness Interest Group (2006). Mindfulness-based psychotherapies: A review of conceptual foundations, empirical evidence and practical considerations. *Australian & New Zealand Journal of Psychiatry, 40*(4), 285–294. https://doi.org/10.1080/j.1440-1614.2006.01794.x

Mensink-Ypma, M. (1990). *Broddelen en leerstoornissen: Aspecten van broddelen en leermoeilijkheden, visie op behandeling* (2nd ed.). Bohn Stafleu van Loghum.

Mensink-Ypma, M. (1990). *Cluttering and learning disabilities.* Bohn Stafleu van Loghum

Menzies, R.G., Onslow, M., Packman, A., & O'Brian, S. (2009). Cognitive behavior therapy for adults who stutter: A tutorial for speech-language pathologists. *Journal of Fluency Disorders, 34*(3), 187–200.

Merwe, A. van der & Steyn, M. (2018). Model-driven treatment of childhood apraxia of speech: Positive effects of the speech motor learning approach. *American Journal of Speech-Language Pathology*, 27(1), 37–51. https://doi.org/10.1044/2017_AJSLP-15-0193

Miller, J.F., Leddy, M.G., & Leavitt, L.A. (1999). *Improving the communication of people with Down syndrome*. Paul H. Brookes Publishing Company.

Missulovin, L. (2002). *Patomorphos of stuttering: Change in picture of the onset and development of stuttering: Specifics of the correctional work*. Souz.

Miyamoto, S. (2011). Assessment and intervention of Japanese children exhibiting possible cluttering. In D. Ward & K. Scaler Scott (eds.), *Cluttering: A handbook of research, intervention and education* (pp. 198–210). Psychology Press.

Miyamoto, S., Hayasaka, K., & Shapiro, D. (2007). An examination of the checklist for possible cluttering in Japan. In J. Au-Yeung & M. Leahy (eds.), *Research, treatment, and self-help in fluency disorders: New horizons* (pp. 279–283). Paper presented at the International Fluency Association.

Mullet, C.F. (1971). 'An arte to make the dumbe speake, the deafe to heare': A seventeenth century goal. *Journal of the History of Medicine and Allied Sciences*, 26(2), 123–140.

Myers, F. L. (1992). Cluttering: A synergistic framework. In F. L. Myers & K. O. St. Lous (Eds.), Cluttering: A clinical perspective (pp. 71–84). Klbworth, Great Britain: Far Communications.

Myers, F., Bakker, K., Cook, S., Reichel, I., St. Louis, K., van Zaalen, Y. (2018). A clinical conceptualization of cluttering. International Cluttering Association, https://drive.google.com/file/d/12ciGPFrQZkLlUlmRRhIMwm5IcGSjJehp/view

Myers, F.L., & Bradley, C.L. (1992). Clinical management of cluttering from a synergistic framework. In F.L. Myers & K.O. St. Louis (eds.), *Cluttering: A clinical perspective* (pp. 85–105). FAR Communications.

Myers, F.L., & St. Louis, K.O. (1992). *Cluttering: A clinical perspective*. FAR Communications.

Myers, F.L., & St. Louis, K.O. (2007). *Cluttering* [dvd]. The Stuttering Foundation.

Myers, F.L. (1996). Annotations of research and clinical perspectives on cluttering since 1964. *Journal of Fluency Disorders*, 21, 187–200.

Myers, F.L. (2011). Treatment of cluttering: A cognitive-behavioral approach centered on rate control. In D. Ward & K. Scaler Scott (eds.), *Cluttering: A handbook of research, intervention and education* (pp. 152–174). Psychology Press.

Nash, H.M., & Snowling, M.J. (2008). Semantic and phonological fluency in children with Down syndrome: Atypical organization of language or less efficient retrieval strategies? *Cognitive Neuropsychology*, 25(5), 690–703.

Neumann, K. (2019). Speech fluency disorders in childhood and adolescence. *HNO*, 67(7), 547–560. https://doi.org/10.1007/s00106-019-0694-7

Nijland, L. (2003). *Developmental apraxia of speech: Deficits in phonetic planning and motor programming* [Doctoral dissertation]. Katholieke Universiteit Nijmegen.

Nijland, L. (2009). Speech perception in children with speech output disorders. *Clinical Linguistics & Phonetics*, 23(3), 222–239.

Ohman, R. (2000). Fear and anxiety: Evolutionary, cognitive, and clinical perspectives. In M. Lewis & J.M. Haviland-Jones (eds.), *Handbook of emotions* (2nd ed.). (pp. 573–593). Guilford Press.

Oliva, F., Malandrone, F., di Girolamo, G., Mirabella, S., Colombi, N., Carletto, S., & Ostacoli, L. (2021). The efficacy of mindfulness-based interventions in attention-deficit/hyperactivity disorder beyond core symptoms: a systematic review, meta-analysis, and meta-regression. *Journal of Affective Disorders*, 292, 475–486. https://doi.org/10.1016/j.jad.2021.05.068

Olsthoorn, N.M. (2007). *Relationships between grammatical encoding and decoding: An experimental psycholinguistic study* [Doctoral dissertation]. Universiteit Leiden, Faculteit der Sociale Wetenschappen.

Op 't Hof, J., & Uys, I. (1974). A clinical delineation of tachyphemia (cluttering): A case of dominant inheritance. *South African Medical Journal*, 48(38), 1624–1628.

Otto, F.M., & Yairi, E. (1975). An analysis of the speech dysfluencies in Down's syndrome and in normally intelligent subjects. *Journal of Fluency Disorders*, 1(4), 26–32.

Overvelde, A., & Hulstijn, W. (2011). Handwriting development in grade 2 and grade 3 primary school children with normal, at risk, or dysgraphic characteristics. *Research in Developmental Disabilities*, 32(2), 540–548. https://doi.org/10.1016/j.ridd.2010.12.027

ParkinsonNL. (n.d.). *Symptomen*. www.parkinson.nl/over-parkinson/symptomen

Perelló, J. (1970). Tachyphemia: A clinical contribution. *Folia Phoniatrica et Logopaedica*, 22(4), 381–382.

Pindzola, R.H., Jenkins, M.M., & Lokken, K.J. (1989). Speaking rates of young children. *Language, Speech, and Hearing Services in Schools*, 20(2), 133–138.

Pitluk, N. (1982). Aspects of the expressive language of cluttering and stuttering school children. *South African Journal of Communication Disorders*, 29, 77–84.

Preus, A. (1972). Stuttering in Down's Syndrome. *Scandinavian Journal of Educational Research*, 16(1), 89–104. https://doi.org/10.1080/0031383720160106

Preus, A. (1981). *Identifying subgroups of stuttering*. Universitetsforlaget.

Preus, A. (1996). Cluttering upgraded. *Journal of Fluency Disorders*, 21, 349–358.

Proctor, A, Yairi, E., Duff, M.C., & Zhang, J. (2008). Prevalence of stuttering in African American preschoolers. *Journal of Speech, Language, and Hearing Research*, 51(6), 1465–1479. https://doi.org/10.1044/1092-4388(2008/07-0057)

Quené, H. (2011). Are we speaking faster than before? In W. Zonneveld, H. Quené & W.F.L. Heeren (eds.), *Sound and sounds: Studies presented to M.E.H. (Bert) Schouten on the occasion of his 65th birthday* (pp. 161–171). UiL-OTS.

Rapoport, M., Reekum, R. van & Mayberg, M.D. (2000). The role of the cerebellum in cognition and behavior: A selective review. *The Journal of Neuropsychiatry and Clinical Neurosciences*, 12(2), 193–198.

Reichel, I.K., & Bakker, K. (2009). Global landscape of cluttering. *Perspectives on Fluency and Fluency Disorders*, 19(2), 62–66.

Reichel, I.K., & Draguns, J. (2011). International perspectives on perceiving, identifying, and managing cluttering. In D. Ward & K. Scaler Scott (eds.), *Cluttering: A handbook of research, intervention and education* (pp. 263–279). Psychology Press.

Reichel, I.K., & St. Louis, K.O. (2007). Mitigating negative stereotyping of stuttering in a fluency disorders class. In J. Au-Yeung & M. Leahy (eds.), *Research, treatment, and self-help in fluency disorders: New horizons* (pp. 236–244). Paper presented at the International Fluency Association.

Reichel, I.K. (2007). *Emotional intelligence and stuttering intervention*. Paper presented at the 10th International Stuttering Awareness Day Online Conference. Retrieved from http://www.mnsu.edu/comdis/isad10/papers/reichel10.html

Reichel, I.K. (2010). Treating the person who clutters and stutters. In K. Bakker, L. Raphael & F. Myers (eds.), *Proceedings of the First World Conference on Cluttering* (pp. 99–108). International Fluency Association.

Reichel, I.K., Bakker, K., & Myers, F. (2010). *The worldwide panorama of cluttering: Non-Western countries*. Paper presented at the International Cluttering Online Conference. Retrieved from http://www.mnsu.edu/comdis/ica1/papers/reichel1c.html

Reichel, I.K., Scaler Scott, K., & Zaalen, Y. van (2012, November). *Tribute to international partnership in research and education in cluttering.* Paper presented at the convention of the American Speech-Language-Hearing Association, Atlanta.

Reichel, I.K., St. Louis, K.O., & Zaalen, Y. van (2013, September). *Emotional intelligence training for speech-language pathologists.* Paper presented at the Fourth International Congress on Emotional Intelligence, New York.

Renfrew, C. (1997). *The Renfrew Language Scales: Bus story test: A test of narrative speech.* Speechmark.

Riley, G.D., & Riley, J. (1985). *Oral motor assessment and treatment: Improving syllable production.* PRO-ED.

Riley, G.D. (2009). *SSI-4: Stuttering Severity Instrument for children and adults* (4th ed.). PRO-ED.

Rodero, E. (2012). Stimulating the imagination in a radio story: The role of presentation structure and the degree of involvement of the listener, *Journal of Radio & Audio Media*, 19(1), 45–60.

Rubin, N., & Henderson, S.E. (1982). Two sides of the same coin: Variations in teaching methods and failure to learn to write. *Special Education: Forward Trends*, 9(4), 17–24.

Rusz, J., Tykalova, T., Ramig, L.O., & Tripoliti, E. (2021). Guidelines for speech recording and acoustic analyses in dysarthrias of movement disorders. *Movement Disorders*, 36(4), 803–814.

Sasisekaran, J., De Nil, L., Smyth, R., & Johnson, C. (2006). Phonological encoding in the silent speech of persons who stutter. *Journal of Fluency Disorders, 31*(1), 1–21.

Scaler Scott, K., & Ward, D. (2013). *Managing cluttering: A comprehensive guidebook of activities.* PRO-ED.

Scaler Scott, K. (2008). *A comparison of disfluency and language in matched children with Asperger's disorder, children who stutter, and controls during an expository discourse task* [Doctoral dissertation]. University of Louisiana.

Scaler Scott, K. (2011). Cluttering and autism spectrum disorders. In D. Ward & K. Scaler Scott (eds.), *Cluttering: A handbook of research, intervention and education* (pp. 115–133). Psychology Press.

Scaler Scott, K., Grossman, H., Abendroth, K.J., Tetnowski, J.A., & Damico, J.S. (2007). Asperger syndrome and attention deficit disorder: Clinical disfluency analysis. In J. Au-Yeung & M. Leahy (eds.), *Research, treatment, and self-help in fluency disorders: New horizons* (pp. 273–278). International Fluency Association.

Scaler Scott, K., Sønsterud, H., & Reichel, I. (2022). Cluttering: Etiology, Symptomatology, Identification, and Treatment. In P. Zebrowski, J. Anderson, & E. Conture (Eds.), *Stuttering: Characteristics, Assessment, and Treatment* (4th ed.). New York, N.Y: Thieme Medical Publishers.

Scharfenaker, S., & Stackhouse, T. (2012). *Strategies for day-to-day-life.* Retrieved from www.fragilex.org/2012/support-and-resources/strategies-for-day-to-day-life

Schneider, D.J. (2004). *The psychology of stereotyping.* Guilford Press.

Schnell, A. (2013). *Prävalenz von Poltersymptomen bei deutschen Kindern* [Bachelor thesis]. Zuyd University of Applied Sciences.

Scott, K.S., & Cummings, L. (2017). Research in clinical pragmatics. In L. Cummings (eds.), *Stuttering and cluttering* (pp. 471–490). Springer International Publishing.

Scott, K.S. (2020). Cluttering symptoms in school-age children by communicative context: a preliminary investigation. *International Journal of Speech-Language Pathology*, 22(2), 174–183. https://doi.org/10.1080/17549507.2019.1637020

Scripture, E.W. (1912). *Stuttering and lisping.* Macmillan.

Seeman, M. (1965). *Sprachstörungen bei Kindern*. Volk und Gesundheit.

Seeman, M. (1970). Relation between motorics of speech and general motor ability in clutterers. *Folia Phoniatrica et Logopaedica, 22*(4), 376–380.

Shapiro, D. (2011). *Stuttering intervention: A collaborative journey to fluency freedom* (2nd ed.). PRO-ED.

Shields, L. (2010). *Treating cluttered speech in a child with autism: Case study*. [Paper presented at the annual convention of the American Speech-Language-Hearing Association.] Philadelphia, PA.

Shklovsky, V.M. (1994). *Stuttering*. Moscow University Press.

Shriberg, L.D. (2003). Diagnostic markers for child speech-sound disorders: Introductory comments. *Clinical Linguistics and Phonetics, 17*(7), 501–505.

Simkins, L. (1973). Cluttering. In B.B. Lahey (ed.), *The modification of language behavior* (pp. 178–217). Charles C. Thomas.

Skodda, S., & Schlegel, U. (2008). Speech rate and rhythm in Parkinson's disease. *Movement Disorders, 23*(7), 985–992.

Smith, A., Goffman, L., Zelaznik, H.N., Ying, G., & McGillem, C. (1995). Spatiotemporal stability and patterning of speech movement sequences. *Experimental Brain Research, 104*(3), 493–501.

St. Louis, K.O., & Hinzman, A.R. (1986). Studies of cluttering: Perceptions of cluttering by speech-language pathologists and educators. *Journal of Fluency Disorders, 11*(2), 131–149.

St. Louis, K.O., & McCaffrey, E. (2005, November). *Public awareness of cluttering and stuttering: Preliminary results*. Poster presented at the annual convention of the American Speech-Language-Hearing Association, San Diego, CA.

St. Louis, K.O., & Myers, F.L. (1997). Management of cluttering and related fluency disorders. In R. Curlee & G. Siegel (eds.), *Nature and treatment of stuttering: New directions* (pp. 313–332). Allyn & Bacon.

St. Louis, K.O., & Rustin, L. (1996). Professional awareness of cluttering. In F.L. Myers & K.O. St. Louis (eds.), *Cluttering: A clinical perspective* (pp. 23–35). Singular.

St. Louis, K.O., & Schulte, K. (2011). Defining cluttering: The lowest common denominator. In D. Ward & K. Scaler Scott (eds.), *Cluttering: A handbook of research, intervention and education* (pp. 233–253). Psychology Press.

St. Louis, K.O. (1992). On defining cluttering. In F.L. Myers & K.O. St. Louis (eds.), *Cluttering: A clinical perspective* (pp. 37–53). FAR Communications.

St. Louis, K.O. (1996). A tabular summary of cluttering subjects in the special edition. *Journal of Fluency Disorders, 21*, 337–344.

St. Louis, K.O. (2011). The public opinion survey of human attributes-stuttering (POSHA-S): summary framework and empirical comparisons. *Journal of Fluency Disorders, 36*(4), 256–261.

St. Louis, K.O. (2013, September). *International Project on Attitudes Toward Human Attributes (IPATHA)*. Paper presented at the Stuttering Attitudes Research Symposium, Morgantown, WV. www.stutteringattitudes.com

St. Louis, K.O., Filatova, Y., Coşkun, M., Topbaş, S., Özdemir, S., Georgieva, D., McCaffrey, E., & George, R.D. (2010). Identification of cluttering and stuttering by the public in four countries. *International Journal of Speech-Language Pathology, 12*(6), 508–519.

St. Louis, K.O., Filatova, Y., Coşkun, M., Topbaş, S., Özdemir, S., Georgieva, D., McCaffrey, E., & George, R.D. (2011). Public attitudes toward cluttering. In E.L. Simon (eds.), *Psychology of stereotypes* (pp. 81–113). Nova Science.

St. Louis, K.O., Hinzman, A.R., & Hull, F.M. (1985). Studies of cluttering: Disfluency and language measures in young possible clutterers and stutterers. *Journal of Fluency Disorders, 10*(3), 151–172.

St. Louis, K.O., Myers, F.L., Bakker, K., & Raphael, L.J. (2007). Understanding and treating cluttering. In E. Conture & R. Curlee (eds.), *Stuttering and other fluency disorders* (3rd ed.) (pp. 297–325). Thieme.

St. Louis, K.O., Myers, F.L., Cassidy, L., Michael, A., Penrod, S., Litton, B., Olivera, J., & Brodsky, E. (1996). Efficacy of delayed auditory feedback for treating cluttering: Two case studies. *Journal of Fluency Disorders*, 21(3–4), 305–314.

St. Louis, K.O., Raphael, L.J., Myers, F.L., & Bakker, K. (2003). Cluttering updated. *The ASHA Leader*, 18(4–5), 20–22.

Stansfield, J. (1990). Prevalence of stuttering and cluttering in adults with mental handicaps. *Journal of Mental Deficiency Research*, 34(4), 287–307.

Starkweather, C.W. (1987). *Fluency and stuttering*. Prentice-Hall.

Steinberg Lowe, M., & Buchwald, A. (2017). The impact of feedback frequency on performance in a novel speech motor learning task. *Journal of Speech, Language, and Hearing Research*, 60(6S), 1712–1725. https://doi.org/10.1044/2017_JSLHR-S-16-0207

Stipancic, K.L., Kuo, Y.-L., Miller, A., Ventresca, H.M., Sternad, D., Kimberley, T.J., & Green, J.R. (2021). The effects of continuous oromotor activity on speech motor learning: Speech biomechanics and neurophysiologic correlates. *Experimental Brain Research*, 239, 3487–3505. https://doi.org/10.3389/fnins.2018.00683

Stoel-Gammon, C. (2001). Down syndrome phonology: Developmental patterns and intervention strategies. *Down Syndrome Research and Practice*, 7(3), 93–100.

Stourneras, E.F. (1980). Stotteren bij kinderen. In C.H. Waar (eds.), *Stem-, spraak- en taalstoornissen bij kinderen* (pp. 65–95). Stafleu.

Sturm, J. A., & Seery, C. H. (2007). Speech and articulatory rates of school-age children in conversation and narrative contexts. *Language, Speech, and Hearing Services in Schools*, 38, 47–59.

Taylor, H., & Vestergaard, M.D. (2022). Developmental dyslexia: Disorder or specialization in exploration? *Frontier Psychology*, 13. https://doi.org/10.3389/fpsyg.2022.889245

Terband, H., Zaalen, Y. van, & Maassen, B. (2013). Lateral jaw stability in adults, children, and children with developmental speech disorders. *Journal of Medical Speech-Language Pathology*, 20(4), 112–118.

Tetnowski, J.A., & Douglass, J. (2011). Cluttering in the academic curriculum. In D. Ward & K. Scaler Scott (eds.), *Cluttering: A handbook of research, intervention and education* (pp. 280–296). Psychology Press.

Thacker, A., & Austen, S. (1996). Cluttered communication in a deafened adult with autistic features. *Journal of Fluency Disorders*, 21, 271–279.

Thyme-Frøkjær, K., & Frøkjær-Jensen, B. (2004). *De Accentmethode: Een stemtherapie in theorie en praktijk*. Pearson.

Tiger, R.J., Irvine, T.L., & Reis, R.P. (1980). Cluttering as a complex of learning disabilities. *Language, Speech, and Hearing Services in Schools*, 11(1), 3–14.

Van Borsel, J., & Tetnowski, J.A. (2007). Fluency disorders in genetic syndromes. *Journal of Fluency Disorders*, 32(4), 279–296.

Van Borsel, J., & Vandermeulen, A. (2008). Cluttering in Down syndrome. *Folia Phoniatrica et Logopaedica*, 60(6), 312–317.

Van Borsel, J., & Vanryckeghem, M. (2000). Dysfluency and phonic tics in Tourette syndrome: A case report. *Journal of Communication Disorders*, 33(3), 227–239.

Van Borsel, J. (1996). Articulation in Down's syndrome adolescents and adults. *International Journal of Language & Communication Disorders*, 31(4), 415–444.

Van Borsel, J. (2011). Cluttering and Down syndrome. In D. Ward & K. Scaler Scott (eds.), *Cluttering: A handbook of research, intervention and education* (pp. 90–99). Psychology Press.

Van Borsel, J., Dor, O., & Rondal, J. (2008). Speech fluency in fragile X syndrome. *Clinical Linguistics and Phonetics, 22*(1), 1–11.

Van Riper, C. (1970). Stuttering and cluttering: The differential diagnosis. *Folia Phoniatrica et Logopaedica, 22*(4), 347–353.

Van Riper, C. (1982). *The nature of stuttering.* Prentice-Hall.

Verhoeven, J., Pauw, G., & Kloots, H. (2004). Speech rate in a pluricentric language: A comparison between Dutch in Belgium and the Netherlands. *Language and Speech, 47*(3), 297–308.

Voelker, C.H. (1935). The prevention of cluttering. *The English Journal, 24*(10), 808–810.

Wallen, M., Bonney, M.A., & Lennox, L. (1996). Handwriting Speed Test. *Australian Occupational Therapy Journal, 53*(2), 141.

Ward, D., & Scaler Scott, K. (2011). *Cluttering: A handbook of research, intervention and education.* Psychology Press.

Ward, D. (2004). Cluttering, speech rate and linguistic deficit: A case report. In A. Packman, A. Meltzer & H.F.M. Peters (eds.), *Theory, research and therapy in fluency disorders. Proceedings of the 4th World Congress on Fluency Disorders, Montreal, Canada* (pp. 511–516). Nijmegen University Press.

Ward, D. (2011). Scope and constraint in the diagnosis of cluttering: Combining two perspectives. In D. Ward & K. Scaler Scott (eds.), *Cluttering: a handbook of research, intervention and education* (pp. 254–263). Psychology Press.

Ward, D. (2018). *Stuttering and cluttering: Frameworks for understanding and treatment.* Psychology Press.

Ward, D., Connally, E.L., Pliatsikas, C., Bretherton-Furness, J., & Watkins, K.E. (2015). The neurological underpinnings of cluttering. Some initial findings. *Journal of Fluency Disorders, 43*, 1–16.

Weiss, D.A. (1964). *Cluttering.* Prentice-Hall.

Weiss, D.A. (1968). Cluttering: Central language imbalance. *Pediatric Clinics of North America, 15*, 705–720.

Weiss, M.G., & Ramakrishna, J. (2006). Stigma interventions and research for international health. *The Lancet, 367*(9509), 536–538.

WHO (2007). *International Classification of Functioning, Disability and Health (ICF).* www.who.int/classifications/icf/en/

Wiele, B., & Zückner, H. (2019). Kinesthetically-controlled speech (kcs) for cluttering: Method and program description. *Forum Logopädie, 33*(2), 6–12.

Wilder, D. (1993). Affect, arousal, and stereotyping. In D.M. Mackie & D.L. Hamilton (eds.), *Affect, cognition, and stereotyping: Interactive processes in group perception* (pp. 87–109). Academic Press/Harcourt Brace Jovanovich.

Wilhelm, R. (2020). *Te snel voor woorden: Hoe de ontdekking dat ik niet stotterde maar broddelde mijn leven veranderde.* Big Time Publishers.

Winkelman, C.L. (1990). Broddelen. In W.M. Mensink-Ypma, *Broddelen en leerstoornissen: Aspecten van broddelen en leermoeilijkheden, visie op behandeling* (2nd ed.) (pp. 142–167). Bohn, Scheltema & Holkema.

Winkelman, C.L. (1993). Broddelen: Een verborgen stoornis. *Logopedie en Foniatrie, 6*, 175–179.

Winkelman, C.L. (2006). Terugrekenoefening. In B.W. Bezemer, J. Bouwen & C. Winkelman, *Stotteren: Van theorie naar therapie* (pp. 320–321). Coutinho.

Wolk, L. (1986). Cluttering: A diagnostic case report. *British Journal of Disorders of Communication, 21*(2), 199–207.

Wright, L., & Ayre, A. (2000). *WASSP: Wright & Ayre Stuttering Self-Rating Profile.* Winslow Press.

Yaruss, S., & Quesal, R. (2010). Overall Assessment of the Speaker's Experience of Stuttering: Documenting multiple outcomes in stuttering treatment. *Journal of Fluency Disorders, 31*(2), 90–115.

Yaruss, S., Logan, K., & Conture, E. (1994). Speaking rate and diadochokinetic abilities of children who stutter. *Journal of Fluency Disorders, 19,* 221–222.

Zaalen, Y. van & Bochane, M. (2007). The wallet story. In *Proceedings of the 27th World Congress of the International Association of Logopedists and Phoniatrics (IALP)* (p. 85). Göteborg University Press.

Zaalen, Y. van & Deckers, S.R.J.M. (2015). *Speech and fluency development in young children with Down Syndrome.* Fontys University of Applied Sciences.

Zaalen, Y. van & Dejonckere, P.H. (2010). *Cluttering: A language-based fluency disorder.* Paper presented at the First Online Conference on cluttering. http://www.mnsu.edu/comdis/ica1/papers/yvonne1c.html

Zaalen, Y. van & Reichel, I.K. (2014). Cluttering treatment: Theoretical considerations and intervention planning. *Perspectives on Global Issues in Communication Sciences and Related Disorders, 4*(2), 57–62.

Zaalen, Y. van & Reichel, I.K. (2015). *Cluttering: Current views on its nature, diagnosis, and treatment.* iUniverse.

Zaalen, Y. van & Reichel, I.K. (2017). Prevalence of cluttering in two European countries: A pilot study. *Perspectives of the ASHA Special Interest Groups, 2*(17), 42–49.

Zaalen, Y. van & Reichel, I.K. (2019). Clinical success using the Audio-Visual Feedback training for cluttering. *Perspectives of the ASHA Special Interest Groups, 4*(6), 1589–1594.

Zaalen, Y. van & Reichel, I.K. (2022). Praktijkboek broddelen: Succesvol behandeld. Coutinho.

Zaalen, Y. van & Strangis, D. (2021). *An adolescent confronted with cluttering: the story of Johan,* Paper presented at the International Conference on Stuttering, IV edition, 14–16th October 2021.

Zaalen, Y. van & Wanseele, B. van (2012). *Cluttering and Parkinson: Kinematic similarities and differences.* Paper presented at the European CPLOL Congress, Den Haag.

Zaalen, Y. van & Winkelman, C. (2009). *Broddelen: Een (on)begrepen stoornis.* Coutinho.

Zaalen, Y. van & Winkelman, C. (2014). *Broddelen: Een (on)begrepen stoornis* (2nd ed.). Coutinho.

Zaalen, Y. van (2009). *Cluttering identified: Differential diagnostics between cluttering, stuttering and learning disability* [Doctoral dissertation]. Universiteit van Utrecht.

Zaalen, Y. van (2010). *Assessment of reading and writing: Consequences for speech therapy in fluency disorders.* Paper presented at the European Symposium on Fluency Disorders, Antwerpen.

Zaalen, Y. van (2011). *Differential diagnostics between cluttering and stuttering: How to do it.* Workshop presented at the Ninth Oxford Disfluency Conference, Oxford.

Zaalen, Y. van, Cook, S., Elings, J., & Howell, P. (2011). *Screening phonological accuracy: Effects of articulatory rate on phonological encoding.* Poster presented at the Speech Motor Conference, Groningen.

Zaalen, Y. van, Deckers, S., Dirven, C., Kaiser, C., Kemenade, P. van & Terhoeve, A. (2012). *Prevalence of cluttering in a school-aged population.* Seminar presented at the Seventh World Congress on Fluency Disorders. International Fluency Association, Tours.

Zaalen, Y. van, Mulderij, M., & Deckers, S. (2020). *Interprofessioneel communiceren in zorg en welzijn.* Coutinho.

Zaalen, Y. van, Myers, F., Ward, D., & Bennett, E. (2008). *The cluttering assessment protocol*. Retrieved from http://associations.missouristate.edu/ICA/

Zaalen, Y. van, Ward, D., Nederveen, A.J., Lameris, J.L., Wijnen, F., & Dejonckere, P.H. (2009e). *Cluttering and stuttering: Different disorders and differing functional neurologies*. Paper presented at the Sixth World Congress on Fluency Disorders, Rio de Janeiro.

Zaalen, Y. van, Wijnen, F., & Dejonckere, P.H. (2009). A test of speech motor control on word level productions: The SPA Test (Screening Pittige Articulatie). *International Journal of Speech and Language Pathology, 11*(1), 26–33.

Zaalen, Y. van, Wijnen, F., & Dejonckere, P.H. (2009b). Language planning disturbances in children who clutter or have learning disabilities. *International Journal of Speech and Language Pathology, 11*(6), 496–508.

Zaalen, Y. van, Wijnen, F., & Dejonckere, P.H. (2009c). Differential diagnostics between cluttering and stuttering: Part one: Speech and language characteristics. *Journal of Fluency Disorders, 34*(3), 137–146.

Zaalen, Y. van, Wijnen, F., & Dejonckere, P.H. (2009d). Differential diagnostics between cluttering and stuttering: Part two: The Predictive Cluttering Inventory-Dutch revised. *Journal of Fluency Disorders, 34*(3), 147–154.

Zaalen, Y. van, Wijnen, F., & Dejonckere, P.H. (2011a). Cluttering and learning disability. In D. Ward & K. Scaler Scott (eds.), *Cluttering: A handbook of research, intervention and education* (pp. 100–114). Psychology Press.

Zaalen, Y. van, Wijnen, F., & Dejonckere, P.H. (2011b). Cluttering assessment: Rationale, tasks and interpretation. In D. Ward & K. Scaler Scott (eds.), *Cluttering: A handbook of research, intervention and education* (pp. 137–151). Psychology Press.

Zajac, D.J., Harris, A.A., Roberts, J.E., & Martin, G.E. (2009). Direct magnitude estimation of articulation rate in boys with fragile X syndrome. *Journal of Speech, Language, and Hearing Research, 52*(5), 1370–1379.

Index

preadolescence, cluttering in 19
Predictive Cluttering Inventory (PCI) 12, 22
Predictive Cluttering Inventory-revised (PCI-r) 62, 198–201
Preus, A. 12, 119
prevalence of cluttering 10, **11**, 12–13, 15, 36
prognosis 18–19
prosody 187; problems 49
public awareness of cluttering 35–36
Public Opinion Survey of Human Attributes-Experimental (POSHA-E) survey 35–36
pure cluttering 95
PWC *see* people with cluttering (PWC)

Quené, H. 58

random variations in execution 143–144
ratio of disfluencies (RDF) 85, 102, 106
RDF *see* ratio of disfluencies (RDF)
reading: analysis of 202–204; passages 225–226
reading aloud 87–88, 100, 103, 159; diagnostic exercise 79
reading text 159–160; for adult readers 216–217
realistic goals 150–151
recordings 156–157; of the reading 160; video 66–67
recordings and questionnaires, analysis of 82–85; disfluencies 84–85; mean articulatory rate (MAR) 83–84, *84*
Reichel, I.K. 5, 20, 35, 93, 124, 130, 137, 142
relaxation 53, 102, 194
repetitions: part-word 46; phrase 114; sentence 10, 46, 135, 136, 177; word 10, 24, 26, 52, 135, 136, 177, 181
retelling a story 69, 73, 80, 85, 88–89, 162, 207–209; analysis of 202–204
rhythm 50, 187
Riley, G.D. 92
Riley, J. 92
Rubin, N. 52
running speech, feedback in 179–181

Schulte, K. 39, 106
Scott, S. 61
screening phonological accuracy (SPA) 92, 98

Scripture, E.W. 101
Seeman, M. 13, 14
self-evaluation of speech 95
self-identification of a symptom 146
self-management 145
self-monitoring 52
self-observation: schedule 147; schemes 152
self-regulation behavior 159
semantic: paraphasias, higher number of 120; storage system 164
sentence repetitions 10, 46, 135–136, 177
sequencing errors 97
Shin, M.S. 106
short- and long-term therapy impact 129–130
Shriberg, L.D. 39
signal-to-noise ratio 156
Simkins, L. 15
SLD *see* specific learning disabilities (SLD)
SLDF *see* stuttering-like disfluencies (SLDF)
sleep, and motor learning 144
SLI *see* specific language impairment (SLI)
slow speech rate 56, 58; *see also* fast speech rate
slurred speech *see* dysarthria
SMA *see* supplementary motor area (SMA)
SMART criteria 140, 142, 146, 192; acceptable 149–150; measurable 147, 149; realistic 150–151; specific 146–147; time-bound 151
Smith, S. 76
Snowling, M.J. 118
social communication, cluttering impact on 131–132
SPA *see* screening phonological accuracy (SPA)
speaker's perceptions 56
speaking situations 141–143, 158, 222; cluttering symptoms in **141**
specific language impairment (SLI) 100–101
specific learning disabilities (SLD) 96
speech analysis 82–85; using PRAAT software 94–95
speech conditions, analysis of 86; case history 86; reading aloud 87–88;

For Product Safety Concerns and Information please contact our EU
representative GPSR@taylorandfrancis.com Taylor & Francis Verlag GmbH,
Kaufingerstraße 24, 80331 München, Germany

Printed and bound by CPI Group (UK) Ltd, Croydon, CR0 4YY
08/06/2025
01897006-0012